CARCINOMA OF THE BREAST

NEW ENGLAND JOURNAL OF MEDICINE
MEDICAL PROGRESS SERIES

CARCINOMA OF THE BREAST

A Decade of New Results with Old Concepts

FRANCIS D. MOORE, M.D.
MOSELEY PROFESSOR OF SURGERY, HARVARD MEDICAL SCHOOL;
SURGEON-IN-CHIEF, PETER BENT BRIGHAM HOSPITAL

STEVEN I. WOODROW, M.D.
ASSISTANT RESIDENT IN SURGERY,
PETER BENT BRIGHAM HOSPITAL

MENELAOS A. ALIAPOULIOS, M.D.
INSTRUCTOR IN SURGERY, HARVARD MEDICAL SCHOOL;
JUNIOR ASSOCIATE IN SURGERY,
PETER BENT BRIGHAM HOSPITAL

RICHARD E. WILSON, M.D.
ASSISTANT PROFESSOR OF SURGERY,
HARVARD MEDICAL SCHOOL; ASSOCIATE IN SURGERY,
PETER BENT BRIGHAM HOSPITAL

LITTLE, BROWN AND COMPANY
BOSTON

THIS MONOGRAPH FIRST APPEARED AS A MEDICAL PROGRESS REPORT IN THE NEW ENGLAND JOURNAL OF MEDICINE.

Published in Great Britain
by J. & A. Churchill Ltd., London

British Standard Book No. 7000 0128 x

PRINTED IN THE UNITED STATES OF AMERICA

To OUR PATIENTS

Those women challenged in the
prime of life by
breast cancer

PREFACE

F ROM time to time an institution should review its experience with a given subject and relate it to that of other institutions. Carcinoma of the breast has been studied as an important clinical problem at the Peter Bent Brigham Hospital for over half a century. In 1956, Dr. A. G. Jessiman and Dr. F. D. Moore reported the experience of this hospital in the *New England Journal of Medicine* and in a subsequent monograph published by Little, Brown and Company. The contents of this book appeared in the *New England Journal of Medicine* in August, 1967.

The present Progress Report was written to document the recent experience of this hospital (1954 to 1963) and to compare it with the experience of others as recorded in the literature. An approach to the treatment of all stages of this disease has been formulated as a point of departure for future work and as a base that others may use if they, too, find it suitable for their patients.

We are indebted to many persons, both for assistance in the care of these patients and for the review of material for this summary. We should particularly like to acknowledge our indebtedness to our medical colleagues, Dr. Kendall Emerson, Dr. Thomas C. Hall, Dr. Hans Nevinny, and the late Dr. Leonid S. Snegireff; to our radiologic colleagues, Dr. James B. Dealy, Jr., and Dr. Martin B. Levene; and to the members of the Surgical Staff (many of whom have cared for the patients mentioned here), particularly to Dr. Donald D. Matson and Dr. Somers H. Sturgis, both of whom have been of constant assistance in dealing with several of the problems of late cancer. Acknowledgment is also made to Mrs. Katherine MacDonald, record librarian for the Breast Tumor Group, Mrs. Donald Height and Miss Carole Krysiak for stenographic assistance, and Miss Regene Gronich and Miss Elise P. Holladay for technical help. Editorial counseling was provided by Mr. Tuckerman Day.

In addition, we acknowledge the many helpful comments received by the *New England Journal of Medicine* which, when feasible, have been incorporated into this version of the Progress Report.

F. D. M.
S. I. W.
M. A. A.
R. E. W.

Boston

CONTENTS

Contents

THERE can be no doubt of the growing importance of breast cancer. This tumor stands unique as the commonest malignant tumor of middle-aged women, and the leading cause of death in white women in the United States, thirty-nine to fifty-four years of age. No single manifestation of cardiovascular or renal disease, no single infection and no complication of pregnancy or parturition takes such a toll of the mother in her prime.

Twelve years ago, in an effort to improve the care of patients suffering from carcinoma of the breast, a group activity was established at the Peter Bent Brigham Hospital, functioning as a division of the Tumor Clinic. Patients were seen by the consultative group, first at the time of the original diagnosis and sequentially throughout the illness. During the ensuing years (January 1, 1954, to June 30, 1966) 616 patients have been treated for this disease at the Peter Bent Brigham Hospital. With December 31, 1963, as the termination of a ten-year cohort and with follow-up data complete to June 30, 1965, data became available on 498 patients. Of these, 25 were excluded because they were seen for consultation only, and this left a group of 473 patients for analysis and for whom follow-up study was complete.

Introduction

During this past decade many investigators have reported definitive results with the therapeutic procedures introduced since World War II. These include adrenalectomy, hypophysectomy and chemotherapy. In addition, information on the treatment of the primary disease is now available, contrasting simple and radical therapies. The new biochemical discriminants have been introduced and put to trial.

It is the purpose of this review to analyze the experience of this hospital in the light of the current literature, and to formulate a program for the management of patients with breast cancer at all stages of their disease. This book updates previous progress reports in the *New England Journal of Medicine*.[1, 2]

Clinical Material and Literature Cited

Among the 473 patients forming the body of this study, 4 were males. Of the 469 females seen and treated for carcinoma of the breast, 248 presented themselves for their first treatment at this hospital. These are identified as the "PBBH primary cases," although 29 of them had extremely advanced or preterminal disease when they first consulted a doctor. Not all these primary patients were deemed suitable for extensive treatment by local surgery of any type; 167 underwent radical mastectomy. There were 3 hospital deaths in this primary group. A total of 135 of the 245 survivors remained free of their carcinoma of the breast, at least for this follow-up period (two to ten years), or died of other causes during that time.

In addition, a total of 221 patients were referred here for treatment of their secondary disease, having undergone primary treatment elsewhere. Of these, 213 actually had recurrent or metastatic carcinoma of the breast, and the patients of this group are designated as the "referred secondary cases." To these 213 patients are added the 110 PBBH primaries who later had recurrences, making a total of 323 patients treated for secondary disease during this ten-year period.*

Of this group of 473 patients treated for breast cancer, 342 are now dead; 131 were alive at the time the study period was closed, with follow-up data in all. Of those who died, 45 died of other diseases, and 297 succumbed to their breast cancer.†

Throughout this decade, treatment of the primary disease has changed but little on this surgical service. Before the start of the study the indications for radical surgery had already been restricted to clinical classes A and B. Increasing use of postoperative irradiation is evident, and supervoltage therapy has become available only in the last few years. The experience with hypophysectomy and adrenalectomy has been gathered entirely during this period, and now includes a total of 163 patients in two sequential series, one of 77 hypophysectomies, and the other of 86 adrenalectomies, carried out by the same surgeons and with follow-up examinations by the same group in identical settings. The extensive use of corticosteroids and of 5-fluorouracil has likewise arisen during this time.

---

* An additional small group of 32 patients in which adrenalectomy has been performed since the close of the study cohort is included in certain of the tables to update the mortality and morbidity for this operation.

† Clinical information and laboratory data on these patients have been analyzed in collaboration with the Biomathematics Division, with the use of standard data-processing methods. We are indebted to Dr. Anthony F. Bartholomay and Dr. Paul S. Levy for advice and assistance throughout.

CARCINOMA OF THE BREAST

1

PREVALENCE, EPIDEMIOLOGY,
PREDISPOSITION AND
CASE FINDINGS

THE phrase "biologic predeterminism" has been coined to present an essentially nihilistic view toward the treatment of cancer: "It makes no difference how you find it, when you treat it, or how you treat it when you find it, the result is predetermined by some inner biologic property of the tumor." In carcinoma of the breast nothing could be further from the case. There is a clear correlation of five-year and ten-year survivals with the size of the tumor, and a partial correlation with location and histologic type, but above all with the extent of lymph-node involvement.[3-5] If one acknowledges that the passage of time is required for a tumor to progress from its initial focus to lymph-node metastasis, one must also accept the corollary that early diagnosis presents the patient with the greatest likelihood of survival: a localized tumor without spread.

Incidence and Prevalence

The incidence and prevalence of this disease is now well established for the United States.[6-8] The age-adjusted incidence rate of cancer for women is 245 cases

1

per 100,000 population per year, with a cancer mortality rate of 133, and a ratio of incidence to mortality of 1.85. In white women the fraction of this total cancer incidence traceable to the breast is close to 25 per cent (60 new cases per 100,000 females per year). Approximately one-quarter of the female population has a lifetime probability of cancer developing in any site, and approximately one-quarter of these will be breast cancers.

Predisposition and the Familial Trend

The genetic soil in which this disease arises has been explored extensively in the last decade by studies of mother-daughter, sibling-pair, patient-aunt and child-suckling relationships.[9-18] From these studies certain generalities emerge: mothers of patients with this disease have a 3 per cent likelihood of developing carcinoma of the breast within a few years of observation of the initial case, sisters about a 10 per cent likelihood, and daughters about a 7 per cent likelihood. One set of data shows early morbid risk as high as 28 per cent among married daughters of patients with this disease, and as high as 13 per cent among sisters. Both Woolf[14] and Anderson et al.[16] found that the hereditary tendency is for breast cancers specifically, and not merely for malignant tumors in general.

These data clearly indicate the advisability of frequent examinations, together with mammograms, of the patient's female relatives. Anderson et al.[16] (1958) have been among the few to put this lesson to work. The same concern applies to the remaining breast after mastectomy for cancer: in approximately 10 per cent of patients surviving for more than three years the lesion will develop in the opposite breast.

2

Nursing

An epidemiologic correlation with the avoidance of nursing encounters statistical difficulty because the disease is so common in the upper-class white population, in which nursing is so rare. In a recent study by Salber and Feinleib,[9] it was found that 22 per cent of 2233 women in Boston, Brookline and Newton, Massachusetts, attempted breast feeding, but only 5 per cent breast-fed their babies for six months or more. Social class and educational status were found to be the most important variables; the wives of students exhibited the highest incidence of breast feeding (69.3 per cent). Women in the upper economic class breast-fed more frequently (39.8 per cent) than those in the lower classes (13.6 per cent).

In the light of these findings, the nursing histories of the PBBH primary cases are of interest. These patients come from the same geographic area as the subjects studied by Salber and Feinleib.[9] Of the 248 patients seen for primary treatment, a nursing history was obtainable in 229. Of these patients 144, or 63 per cent, had nursed their children for less than two weeks or not at all. Only 61, or 27 per cent, had nursed their children for a total of more than three months. Of the 214 women with an onset of disease under the age of fifty, a nursing history was obtainable in 192, and of these only 36, or 17 per cent, had nursed for over three months.

The data from the PBBH primary cases thus occupy an intermediate position between the two extremes reported by Salber and Feinleib.[9] It is not possible to draw any clear-cut conclusion from them, but the data do indicate that failure to nurse for longer than three months is associated with a higher risk of breast cancer. This association does not establish cause and effect, and must be viewed with due respect for the effects of gravidity and parity on the incidence of the disease.

Endocrine Factors

Endocrine factors in the epidemiology of breast cancer are at least three in number: parity, menarche-menopause and previous oophorectomy.

As for *parity,* nulliparity and nulligravidity increase the risk of breast cancer. It is not known whether marriage and childbearing actually protect a woman against the disease, or whether the women who are somehow ensured against the disease possess some secondary sex characteristic that makes them more apt to marry and bear children. Whatever cause-effect relation ultimately emerges, the statistical correlation remains that the disease is significantly less frequent in married women who have borne children than in single nulliparous women. The data on the PBBH primary cases bear this out to a remarkable extent. A disproportionately large number of these patients (20 per cent) were single women, and a full 34 per cent of them were nulliparous. Yet multiparity alone is little protection against this disease; of the 469 female patients treated 187, or 40 per cent, had 3 or more children.

The *menopause* occupies a unique position in relation to cancer of the breast: the majority of patients seen and treated for this disease are in the group from forty-five to fifty-five years of age. Despite this seeming frequency in the decade of the menopause, corrected curves show that the steadily rising incidence actually levels off for a few years at this time of life before again assuming its sharply rising inflection. Thus, any clinic will see most patients with this disease during the menopausal years, but if a woman survives this high-risk period of her life, she derives little protection from advancing age. The statistical likelihood of her acquiring breast cancer increases steadily with each passing decade.

In the endocrine sphere should be noted the possible, although unproved, adverse effects of oral contraceptives. Five to 10 per cent of patients on oral contraceptives observe an increase in heaviness and discomfort in the breast. In a recent report by Gregg[19] a patient showed galactorrhea with increased pigmentation of the nipples and multiple fibroadenomas in both breasts when she was taking oral contraceptives. The facts indicate merely that oral contraceptives have an impact on breast physiology and anatomy. They do not establish any clear association with breast cancer itself. Whether the upset of normal ovulation and reproductive physiology produced by the contraceptive pills will be followed by an increased incidence of carcinoma of the breast, either from the medicines themselves or from the avoidance of pregnancy, remains to be ascertained. In a young married woman with a positive family history of breast cancer one can hardly support prolonged use of contraceptive pills to avoid pregnancy, lactation and nursing.

In a patient who has had a carcinoma of the breast removed, and in whom further pregnancy is to be avoided for fear of exacerbation of dormant metastases, the oral contraceptive pills are positively contraindicated. Many contain progestins, and others estrogens, both substances that will stimulate the growth of dormant breast metastases. A recent study[20] has shown marked stimulation of advanced breast cancer — as evidenced by acute hypercalcemia — after the administration of a modified progestational agent, medroxy-progesterone acetate (Provera). If pregnancy is to be avoided in such patients, an intrauterine device or some other nonhormonal method of birth control should be used.

Previous oophorectomy appears to reduce the incidence of breast cancer as reported in the study of Mac-Mahon and Feinleib,[21] which shows a significantly lower incidence of prior surgical removal of pelvic genitalia in the breast-cancer group as contrasted with matched controls. There is evidence from the experience at the Peter Bent Brigham Hospital that if this disease develops in a patient who has undergone prior oophorectomy, she then has a significantly worse prognosis. This is demonstrated by the fact that among the 110 patients from the PBBH primary group who later went on to develop the advanced disease, a larger fraction than in any of the other subgroups analyzed had undergone bilateral oophorectomy before the onset of the breast cancer.

Case Findings — Delay Factors, Previous Breast Disease and Biopsy Procedure

Delay factors in diagnosis have an adverse effect on survival, but in most series the overall duration of the tumor can be demonstrated to have an adverse effect only up to about six months. Many patients with tumors that have been present for more than six months show an improved survival over those of somewhat shorter duration, suggesting that some of these delayed tumors are of slower growth potential. This is a phenomenon notable also in carcinoma of the stomach and colon, and is the only detail in the entire epidemiology that might give some support to the concept of biologic predeterminism.

In this clinical material, among 458 cases in which delay factors could be evaluated, there were 282 (62 per cent) in which delay was of little consequence. In 163 patients (38 per cent) there was excessive delay, and in 133 of these (81 per cent) it was directly traceable to patient-based factors. In 30 (19 per cent) there was retrospective recall of a doctor's error.

Most breast cancers are discovered by the patient. Copeland states (in a personal communication) that of 183 patients for whom this information was obtainable, 167 (91 per cent) found the mass themselves. As mentioned above, 80 per cent of the patients in whom delay has occurred have caused it themselves. The most frequent statement is that the lesion was thought to be of little consequence; almost as often the patient thought it might be cancer and was worried lest this suspicion be confirmed.

As for *previous breast disease,* out of 408 patients in whom the presence or absence of previous disease could be determined, there was no history in 296 (73 per cent). In 112 (27 per cent) there was significant previous breast disease, and in 23 of these there had been a previous breast biopsy. The most important point in this area arises when one is dealing with an individual patient who suffers from recurrent, chronic, often painful, lumpy breasts due to chronic cystic mastitis and its several related pathologic entities. Breast cancer can arise in such breasts, and its diagnosis is particularly difficult.

Biopsy procedure must take into consideration the several situations that arise and the several modalities available. The policy used in this hospital is as follows:

Early biopsy should be urged for all patients who state that they have found a lump in the breast and in whom a discrete mass can be felt. This biopsy is best done in the hospital, and should be preceded by the simplest search for metastatic disease, consisting of a film of the chest that also shows the bones of the shoulder girdle and an abdominal film that also shows the bones of the pelvis and upper femora.

Open biopsy should be excisional if possible; needle biopsy is very useful, but is acceptable only if positive. Aspiration of breast cysts for cytologic smear of the aspirate is unacceptable and is not an equivalent to biopsy.

Patients with known benign and recurrent lumps in the breasts (frequently with prior benign biopsy) in whom a new mass is found should be observed again after a six-week interval. At this time the menstrual cycle will be in an alternative phase; only if the lump gets smaller can biopsy be avoided.

Mammography is particularly useful in following the progress of patients with bilateral lumpy breasts before a small carcinoma can frequently be distinguished radiographically from cysts and fibromatous tumors; the radiation dosage is negligible.

In patients with bilateral lumpy breasts who are past the reproductive age and not concerned with cosmetic factors (particularly women with a positive family history for carcinoma) simple mastectomy provides prophylaxis against cancer and a relief from the emotional strain of repeated biopsy.

The age-old fear of delay between biopsy and operation need not be invoked to panic the patient into immediate hospitalization and surgery without suitable study. With either needle biopsy or excisional biopsy, it is almost impossible to demonstrate an adverse effect from a brief interval before operation.

The recent report by Abramson[22] is of particular importance in this regard. He reports his experience with breast biopsy as an outpatient procedure. He could detect no apparent deleterious effect from a delay of up to four days between biopsy and mastectomy. Although our own experience would not recommend breast biopsy as an outpatient procedure, one must expect approximately 6 negative biopsies for each carcinoma found, and everything must be done to simplify the procedure for both patient and hospital.

2

PRIMARY TREATMENT OF THE LOCALIZED DISEASE

FOR the past fifteen or twenty years, there has been an increasing tendency for surgeons to avoid mastectomy in locally advanced cases. This avoidance of radical mastectomy in unfavorable cases marks a distinct advance in the treatment of this disease, and is traceable to the work of many scholars of this subject, but particularly to the studies of Haagensen. He has developed a simple clinical classification of this disease and has emphasized the limitations of radical mastectomy.[23-25]

Haagensen's clinical classification, as employed in the analysis of this disease, should be based solely on the physical and radiologic appearance of the patient. It distinguishes between the limited local tumors (Class A), those with minimal nodal palpable metastases (Class B), locally advanced tumors that are invasive in the breast or excessively metastatic to lymph nodes despite absence of remote metastases (Class C) and finally those with established blood-borne metastases (Class D). This classification provides a dividing line (beyond Class B) where radical mastectomy is of little avail and may shorten life. This classification should not be confused, in its initial presentation or analysis, by subsequent pathologic findings. These should be entered as they become available, and suitably added to the terminology: "clinical Class A, with involved lymph nodes," for example.

In this chapter we recommend a policy for primary treatment of localized breast cancer.

Primary Treatment of Localized Breast Cancer

This policy is based on 5 postulates and involves 5 procedures.

The *postulates* are as follows:

In the first place, mastectomy provides a survival rate of 80 to 90 per cent in patients in clinical Class A whose axillary lymph nodes are negative histologically. No other procedure has been able to compete with this record in the favorable lesions; the finding of one or two involved nodes low in the axilla has little adverse effect on prognosis.

Secondly, dissection and removal of the axillary lymph nodes are essential to provide an adequate specimen for the pathologist, study of which becomes the most important single factor in determining the ultimate prognosis and the details of further treatment.

Thirdly, the most convenient method for removal of the tumor that will, at the same time, provide the pathologist with the axillary specimen for study is the standard radical mastectomy.

Fourthly, given the site and size of the local lesion and the extent of axillary involvement, the involvement of other lymph nodes can then be predicted according to the following scheme, as modified from Haagensen. There is a 30 per cent (or greater) likelihood of apical-axillary or internal-mammary-node involvement if the axillary nodes are more than 2.5 cm. in diameter, in patients in clinical Class B with proved axillary nodal involvement and if the lesion is medial or subareolar.

Finally, when a 30 per cent (or greater) likelihood of apical-axillary involvement or internal mammary involvement has been established it is possible by high-dose, supervoltage irradiation to sterilize unremoved involved nodes in a significant fraction of these patients. Cyclic menstrual activity stimulates residual tumor cells, which can be assumed to be present in 60 per cent of patients with involved nodes; castration prevents this cyclic menstrual activity.

The *procedures* are as follows:

In the first place, early biopsy is essential; lymph nodes are not biopsied unless they are the only presenting manifestation of the disease.

Secondly, patients in clinical Classes A and B are assigned for mastectomy and axillary dissection; patients in clinical Classes C and D are treated as having advanced disease (see below).

Thirdly, for lateral lesions mastectomy combined with axillary dissection is carried out for cure; if the nodes are negative no further treatment is given.

Fourthly, if axillary nodes are positive, postoperative irradiation is given to the axillary, supraclavicular and both internal mammary areas but not to the operative site; with the lesion central or mesial, and regardless of the status of the axillary nodes, irradiation is given as outlined above.

Finally, if the patient is still menstruating or within five years of the spontaneous menopause, surgical castration (oophorectomy) is carried out in patients who receive postoperative irradiation.

The evidence upon which these postulates and procedures are based can conveniently be divided into several groups: general survival data and histologic grading, the controversy between minimal surgery and maximal surgery, the use of postoperative irradiation, the use of postoperative castration, and the use of adjuvant chemotherapy.

General Survival and Histologic Data

In the patients in clinical Class A with negative axillary lymph nodes, the results of mastectomy are so good that with certain favorable histologic types, survival statistics can be superimposed on curves for the rest of the population. It is not surprising that the addition of oophorectomy or postoperative irradiation makes little or no contribution in such favorable cases: one is already dealing with a ceiling survival potential.

This excellent result in a small, highly favorable

group of patients has repeatedly tempted surgeons to simplify therapy, and it has also confused many statistical studies. If a large number of these patients (clinical Class A with negative lymph nodes) are included in a study of postoperative irradiation or castration, they will submerge any potentially significant statistical differences that might exist among treatment groups in which the nodes are involved. It is in the latter group, with nodes involved and prognosis less favorable (about 60 per cent five-year survival for clinical Class B with involved nodes), that a search for improvement in management has been so intense in the past two decades.

A number of interesting studies of the treatment of breast cancer have been reported from universities, teaching hospitals and community groups, in each case relating the therapy and results, at least in part, to the community ecology. Examples are to be found in the studies of Byrd et al.[26] and Moore, Judd and Moore.[27] The studies of Byrd and his associates, like those of Breslow,[28] show that a poorer prognosis obtains in patients in the public wards and from a lower socioeconomic group; the private patients in a university hospital seem to have a higher survival rate. It is probable that the difference in socioeconomic class is related to the stage of the disease when the patient is first seen rather than to any other factor. The data of the California Tumor Registry, used by Dr. Breslow, suggest differences in survival rate even when the data are restricted to cases designated as localized. Byrd and his co-workers[26] demonstrated an improvement in survival rate from mastectomy when it was followed by irradiation therapy in patients with axillary metastases.

The study of Butcher,[29] based on 739 cases analyzed by the method of probits, has shown that, at the extremes, histologic appearance of the tumor is as important as clinical and pathologic staging in determining the results. This is an unusual conclusion for a recent study of breast cancer, and can be reconciled with the experience of others only by its corroboration of the importance of the two ends of the histologic spectrum.

Smithers[4] has made a study of "short survival in early cases and long survival in advanced cases." He agrees that histologic grading has significance, in the sense of predicting early bloodstream involvement. He also agrees that there is no such thing as biologic predeterminism in this disease, and states that "there must be a time in every case when simple mastectomy could effect a cure."

Simple Mastectomy versus Super-radical Mastectomy

The controversy between the advocates of minimal surgery and those of maximal surgery must find its reference point on the middle ground of radical mastectomy.

Using a policy of "mastectomy by exclusion," Haagensen has reported the highest survival rates currently available in the literature. By clinical classification and preliminary lymph-node biopsy, he has been able to identify a group of patients with survival rates as high as 90.6 per cent five years alive and well, free of disease. Haagensen's data scale sharply down from there according to nodal involvement. A representative table of the Haagensen results is shown in the Haagensen and Cooley publication in 1963.[24] The issue with Haagensen's work does not refer to the excellence of his results (having isolated an extremely favorable group for radical mastectomy), but rather to two ancillary considerations. The first is, what does preliminary lymph-node biopsy contribute? Secondly, would there not be a higher cure rate in some patients with positive nodes, if they had received the benefit of mastectomy combined with axillary dissection?

Regarding the first of these questions — the utility of preliminary node biopsy — it is evident from the data of Haagensen (taken together with the information provided by extended radical mastectomy as described below) that it is no longer necessary to carry out preliminary lymph-node biopsy in more than a small fraction of cases. The only lingering justification might lie in a patient with a large mesial lesion, in whom the preliminary finding of an involved axillary lymph node would contraindicate a classic radical mastectomy.

The answer to the second question — whether nodal involvement should preclude mastectomy — rests on the studies of Guttman[30] (referred to below).

Miller[31] attempted to reproduce certain features of the Haagensen procedure. Postoperative radiotherapy was very widely used in these cases, in contrast to Haagensen's practice. The results did not appear to be improved, again because of the statistical impossibility of improving results in a mixed cohort, one moiety of which is large in number and already at a maximal survivorship.

The extremely high cure rate for patients in clinical Class A with negative lymph nodes has stimulated a surgical approach less drastic than radical mastectomy. The proponents of such a view are apt to neglect the important diagnostic contribution made by the products of axillary dissection.

McWhirter[32] was the first revivalist after World War

II to advance the cause of simple mastectomy; as a radiotherapist, he proposed irradiation to deal with lymph nodes, not knowing the extent of their involvement. His reports and those of Ackerman[33] should be consulted in sequence. McWhirter claimed a survival of 53 per cent in an operable group at five years; clearly, this is not a very remarkable result, and is somewhat lower than that claimed by others for radical mastectomy in the Class B group. His operable group included some cases in Class A, and it is surprising that the figure is not higher. Inner-half lesions are unfavorable, since internal-mammary-lymph node involvement is known to be present in 40 to 50 per cent of patients. The 65 per cent five-year survival rate reported for medial lesions treated by simple mastectomy and irradiation is significant for two reasons: because it is a rather high cure rate, and because the mastectomy probably makes little contribution to success. McWhirter was here dealing with the effect of irradiation on internal mammary lymph nodes, and his results are a forerunner of what was later reported by Guttman.[30]

Ackerman's[33] study demonstrates what happens when a pathologist evaluates the surgical results of a radiotherapist. Ackerman found that 13 of McWhirter's patients did not have cancer at all. Three patients later required amputation of an arm, and 220 of the 719 patients had nodes that were later excised or received hormones and other forms of therapy — hardly a control test of any form of treatment. There were 220 patients who had x-ray therapy regardless of the state of the disease, the age of the patient or other factors. Not only was excision of involved nodes used, but likewise stilbestrol and testosterone. Ackerman perceives that the mastectomy probably makes very little contribution to the McWhirter therapy when nodes are involved. He makes the cogent point that McWhirter "has presented no objective evidence of the necessity for simple mastectomy."

Crile[34,35] has advanced a further extension of McWhirter's concept, stating that he favors only the most simplified and minimal approach to the local disease, in some cases little more than a biopsy excision. In his presentations Crile emphasizes the emotional trauma of radical mastectomy, its crippling and its cosmetic price. In one of his recent reports, Crile contrasts patients treated by a surgeon who performed "chiefly simple operations" with those treated by a group of surgeons who performed "chiefly radical ones." There are many hidden subgroups in this study because (like McWhirter before him) Crile frequently abandons his stated program, and if, upon palpating the opened axilla, he encounters swollen nodes, he proceeds to carry out a radical axillary dissection. Approximately 32 of the patients initially thought to have negative axillary lymph nodes were found to have involvement on pathologic examination, and in some of these the axillary dissection was delayed for several weeks or months. This mixture of simple mastectomy with palpation of the axilla, possibly the use of an axillary dissection and possibly a subsequent axillary dissection, with or without irradiation, is no longer a simplified treatment.

In contrast to these advocates of minimal or "simplified" surgery, Urban has been the outstanding proponent of a much more radical approach to the disease. His experience now includes 563 cases;[36] of this entire group, 48 per cent had axillary-lymph-node involvement, and 33.5 per cent had internal-mammary-lymph-node involvement. Reports of his work[37,38] demonstrate two points that are outstanding. In the first place, the expertise developed by Urban and his group enables him to perform an operation involving extensive thoracic dissection with a mortality of only 0.4 per cent. Secondly, his operability criteria are very permissive. In all, 88 per cent of previously untreated primary breast cancers encountered in his clinic have been considered operable. He has a local recurrence rate of only 7.3 per cent and concludes that his salvage rate has been 5 to 10 per cent higher than that anticipated for similar material treated by standard radical mastectomy. At present Urban performs an extended radical operation in about 30 per cent of patients, particularly those with inner-quadrant and central lesions. About 60 per cent of his patients undergo a classic radical, and about 10 per cent a modified radical mastectomy leaving the muscles in place. He uses postoperative radiotherapy when the lymph nodes are involved, and favors total doses in the region of 5000 R, given by supervoltage technics over a protracted period. There was a time when even larger doses were given to his group with positive lymph nodes, but because of bothersome complications, he now advocates the more modest dose.

It is difficult to regard Urban's results as a basis for change in treatment policy for any individual hospital. His five-year survival rates for patients with axillary-lymph-node involvement (around 60 per cent) are grossly in excess of those reported by others. There is no way of contrasting Urban's results when the internal mammary lymph nodes are involved with those of other, lesser procedures because those doing such operations do not really know whether or not the internal mammary lymph nodes are involved (with the exception of Guttman's radiotherapy reports).

Urban's results, when both axillary and internal mammary nodes are involved (about 40 per cent five-year survival) are low enough to suggest that the disease is already blood-borne at that time and that the additional operative procedure is not curing many more patients.

The studies of Kaae and Johansen[39] showed no clear superiority for the super-radical operation in a controlled clinical trial, and the work of Guttman[30,40] suggests that the extended radical operation is rarely required. Kaae and Johansen reported 426 cases divided into two groups and comparable in every respect except for the difference in therapy modality: simple mastectomy plus irradiation versus extended radical mastectomy. Among the 98 patients having simple mastectomy and irradiation and followed for five years, 36 were living and well, as compared with 39 of the 106 who had extended radical mastectomy. The difference, with chance-probability values between 0.1 and 0.2, is not significant.

It is evident from these data that there is little to support the abandonment of mastectomy with axillary dissection in patients in clinical Class A and B. The situation is quite the reverse when nodes are heavily involved, as described below.

Postoperative Irradiation

Several reports on postoperative radiotherapy should be mentioned before we turn to Guttman's work, which appears to answer the most important fundamental question presented by radiotherapy. The reason for disposing of the other reports so briefly is that they are largely inconclusive. Moore and his associates[27] showed a statistically significant improvement in patients with axillary-lymph-node involvement if postoperative radio-therapy was given. Devitt and Beattie[5] observed the least evidence of local recurrence when radical mastectomy was followed by irradiation. Hickey et al.[41] reported no improvement with postoperative irradiation in patients with axillary-lymph-node involvement.

Smith and Smith[42] found a statistically significant improvement when x-ray treatment was given to patients with positive axillary lymph nodes. Lewison and Smith[43] reported a strongly significant improvement at the ten-year level when radiotherapy was given. At five years, the difference was not striking. Butcher and his co-workers[44] brought forth evidence that postoperative radiotherapy had no effect. Like so many other groups, they reported on the use of 250-kv. therapy.

Robbins et al.[45] described two sequential series from Memorial Hospital in New York. One received x-ray therapy, and the other did not, both on a routine basis and without differentiation for nodal involvement. In retrospect, the local recurrence rate in the supraclavicular nodes was significantly less (13 per cent as against 26 per cent) in patients with axillary metastases if they received postoperative x-ray therapy, as contrasted with those who did not. All the other data were identical in the two groups, the patients with negative nodes being analyzed together with all others.

The work of Guttman[30,40] provides important information that has not come from any other surgical-radiologic collaboration. To understand the significance of this contribution, one has to appreciate the setting in which it was carried out: in the same hospital where Haagensen was carrying out "mastectomy by exclusion," Guttman treated the patients who were excluded. Intrinsic in this selection procedure is the fact that a large group of patients must of necessity be excluded for radical mastectomy but who fall into clinical Class A (with positive triple biopsies), Class B or Class C. There are thus, among these patients turned over to Guttman for radiotherapy, many who would look deceptively uncomplicated for radical surgery in the hands of most surgeons.

Each of these patients was treated with extensive supervoltage irradiation. Although five-year survival rates as high as 65 per cent were achieved in some groups and there was an overall salvage competitive with most therapies proposed for such patients, it is notable that Guttman herself would not suggest radiotherapy as the sole method of treatment in a patient with Class A disease and negative nodes.[46]

One may conclude from Guttman's work that supervoltage large-field irradiation at high dose used aggressively can "sterilize" involved nodes in this disease — at least to the five-year survival level. If bloodstream invasion has not yet occurred, one has the remarkable opportunity of achieving a cure with a second modality.

This provides the basis for the recommendation that mastectomy combined with axillary dissection be followed by supervoltage irradiation when the axillary nodes are shown to be involved or when other criteria, as outlined above, indicate that there is a 30 to 50 per cent likelihood of involvement of the apical axillary or internal mammary lymph nodes.*

In postoperative patients with axillary involvement the operative site itself is not irradiated. The areas

* The procedure at this hospital, under the guidance of Dr. James B. Dealy and Dr. Martin Levene, has been to deliver a tissue dose of 4125 rads at a depth of 4 to 5 cm. in 15 treatment sessions, with the use of 6-Mev equipment. The daily increment is 270 rads and the total elapsed time is nineteen to twenty-one days.

treated are bilateral internal mammary nodes, ipsilateral supraclavicular nodes and the apex of the axilla. In this program the incidence of significant complications is in the order of only a few per cent. Radiation esophagitis is the most distressing complication and may become severe enough so that patients go through a period of two or three days of almost complete inability to swallow before they are finally relieved. Asymptomatic radiation fibrosis of the lung apex occurs in a substantial number of patients.

Differences in opinion of the value of postoperative radiotherapy seem likely to persist for many years. Differences in technics account for many varying opinions, and the inclusion of the operative site itself has led to very poor results in the hands of many. Dao and Kovaric[47] have brought forth evidence that local therapy increases the rate of local recurrence in the skin (and ipsilateral lung apex) if the operative site itself is treated. This has not been a part of the routine at this hospital, and we have not seen the phenomenon that he so graphically records.

Castration

The most controversial of the features of treatment policy outlined at the outset of this section is the use of castration in young women with positive nodal involvement. The current evidence on this point remains unconvincing.

The most satisfactory evidence in favor of oophorectomy for patients with involved nodes arises not from the relatively few controlled clinical studies but rather from two completely separate considerations. The first is the fact that of all patients with axillary lymph nodes involved, about half will carry living cancer cells in their bodies after the operation. The second is the demonstration by Pearson et al.[48] that the cyclic estrogenic stimulation of the first half of a normal menstrual cycle is associated with a clearly demonstrable stimulation of the growth of breast cancer. Previous studies here[49,50] indicated that all patients under the age of sixty-five go through a prolonged period when their breast cancer is readily stimulated by estrogens.

Postoperative castration has as its object the removal of this cyclic stimulation of the tumor. This is sometimes called "prophylactic" castration, but it should more appropriately be called "early" castration because, if done in patients in whom the axillary nodes are involved, it is therapeutic rather than prophylactic. In the policy recommended in the foregoing discussion it will be noted that castration is used according to the same considerations holding for postoperative irradiation, and for the same assumption of the continued presence of disease.

Attempts to demonstrate that there is a longer free interval or a better five-year survival rate when early castration is used in patients with positive nodes are few. The article by Smith and Smith[42] is one of the few that appears to show statistically significant improvement. Kennedy and his associates[51,52] disagree with the conclusions of Smith and Smith. In one of their studies he and his co-workers were dealing with a total population of 2908 patients, 296 of whom had oophorectomy at one time or another. Of these, 119 were early oophorectomies and 177 were therapeutic — meaning that they were performed after recurrent disease became visible. In this article no effort is made to separate the early cases according to whether or not axillary lymph nodes were involved. Despite this limitation, their study does show a longer free interval in patients having an early oophorectomy (thirty-eight months versus twenty-one months).

Nissen-Meyer[53] studied oophorectomy versus ovarian irradiation in patients with positive nodes and ovarian irradiation versus no treatment in patients with negative nodes. Paterson and Russell[54] carried out a study of this subject. They administered "a single X-ray treatment delivering a dose of 450 r to each ovary through paired opposing fields of 10-15 cm."* There are no endocrine data, no data on vaginal cytology and no clinical follow-up data to indicate whether or not these patients were effectively castrated by this therapy. The results are inconclusive, but the trend is for improvement in the ovary-irradiated cases whether or not the axillary nodes were involved.

No matter what one's concern is for reduction in the growth potential of the remaining tumor cells, the psychologic and emotional overtones of castration remain a barrier to this procedure. Assuredly, castration should not be offered the patient with a small lateral-quadrant lesion and negative nodes.

The suggestion has been made that oophorectomy should not be carried out early in primary treatment so that it can be "saved until later," when the therapeu-

---

* Dealy[55] points out that the administration of 1600 R to the ovaries over a period of twelve to sixteen days is necessary to suppress estrogen production as demonstrated by subsequent biologic assay. This is approximately equivalent to 800 R in a single administration. This likewise casts doubt on the assertion of Paterson and Russell[54] that they had achieved the endocrine effects of castration with low-dose irradiation. Menstrual periods may have ceased in these patients, but estrogen production must be demonstrated to be reduced by assay or by vaginal cytology before one can assert that such a small dose of x-rays has had the same effect as oophorectomy.

tic response should provide a clear guide to subsequent management. It has now become evident that the oophorectomy response is not a controlling guide to subsequent therapy, and that the choice of timing for oophorectomy should be based on the assumption of the continued presence of disease, and thus hinge upon the local lesion and the extent of nodal involvement rather than other considerations.

Adjuvant Chemotherapy

The administration of cancer chemotherapy during the operative period is based on the finding of cancer cells in the blood at that time. The prognostic significance of such cancer cells remains obscure; their viability and identification has at times been in doubt. In any event, there is little likelihood that transient chemotherapy will materially affect the progress of a disease whose course may last for several decades. It is thus not surprising to find that the adjuvant chemotherapy protocol has thus far failed to show any clear effects.[56]

Primary Treatment of Patients with Locally Advanced Disease When First Seen

The foregoing plan and its supporting data cover the treatment of the early or potentially curable patients in Classes A and B. Policy for those in Classes C and D does not approximate the optimism with which one can approach the early cases.

These patients divide themselves into 2 groups: those still considered by the patient or her doctor to be favorable primary cases, but found on physical examination to be Class C, with a large local lesion, medial location or extensive axillary and supraclavicular nodes; and patients who present themselves to the physician for the first time with remote metastatic disease already present. The latter (Class D) cases should be treated as secondary disease (see below); radiotherapy is all that need be done for the local lesion after the diagnosis has been established by needle biopsy.

It is the patients in Class C — unsuitable for radical mastectomy but with disease still localized to the breast and axilla — who present a problem requiring particular identification and solution. At present the most effective step appears to be local irradiation. Simple mastectomy contributes little to the welfare of these patients unless the breast is very large and pendulous. The radiotherapist might prefer its removal to simplify dosimetry. Under most other circumstances radiotherapy is quite effective for both local disease and local axillary metastases, whereas, by contrast, simple mastectomy will frequently cut through lymph-borne disease and result in local recurrence or intracutaneous spread of a type rarely seen in the absence of surgical attack.

Having dealt with the local disease in Class C by radiotherapy, one can make out an excellent argument for proceeding directly with the therapeutic modalities most effective for secondary disease oophorectomy and adrenalectomy.

3

THE PBBH PRIMARY CASES

DATA from the 248 female patients who presented themselves to this hospital for primary treatment during the period 1954 to 1963 largely corroborate the foregoing conclusions although radical mastectomy was the standard treatment throughout the period, and the policy of avoiding radical surgery in locally advanced cases was becoming established throughout the decade.

In this group of 248 patients, there are follow-up data for periods of five years or longer in 121.* As shown in Table 1, the five-year salvage for all patients presenting primary tumors was 44 per cent, ranging from a high of 78 per cent in the group with no nodes in the specimen, to low residual survival rates in the inoperable cases. Of the patients who presented themselves for treatment, 65 per cent were potentially curable (Classes A or B) when first seen, but only half of these were discovered later to have disease localized to the breast pathologically.

There were 167 radical mastectomies carried out in the ten-year period, with 3 deaths, an operative mortality of 1.8 per cent.

---

* The tables specify patients analyzed from the experience of the entire decade, as contrasted with the group for whom five-year follow-up study is uniform. The criterion of "five years alive and well, free of disease" is employed for survival information. This does not deny the importance of the point, re-emphasized recently by Berg and Robbins,[57] that this cancer, possibly more than any other, requires analysis at intervals of ten, fifteen and twenty years after treatment.

TABLE 1. *Overall Results in PBBH Primary Cases*

Group	Number of Cases	
Total, 1954–1963		248
Total, 1954–1959		121
Clinical Class A	52/121 (43%)	
Clinical Class B	27/121 (22%)	
Clinical Class C	23/121 (19%)	
Clinical Class D	19/121 (16%)	
Death from other causes		15/121 (12%)
All cases at risk for 5-yr. survival		106
5-yr. alive and well, free of disease,* all cases	47/106 (44%)	
Radical mastectomy, with no lymph nodes in specimen		35
Death from other causes	8	
Radical mastectomy, with no lymph nodes, at risk		27
Radical mastectomy, with no lymph nodes, 5-yr. alive and well	21/27 (78%)	
Clinical Classes A and B		79
Death from other causes	10	
Conservative treatment	11	
Radical mastectomy, Classes A and B, at risk		58
Radical mastectomy, Classes A and B, 5-yr. alive and well	41/58 (71%)	
Clinical Classes C and D		42
Death from other causes	2	
Radical mastectomy, Classes C and D, at risk		6
Radical mastectomy, Classes C and D, 5-yr. alive and well	1/6 (17%)	
Conservative operations, Classes C and D, at risk		34
Conservative operations, 5-yr. alive and well	2/34 (6%)	

* In this and subsequent tables, "5-yr. alive and well, free of disease" refers to cases in the 1954–1959 group; designation "2–10 yr. alive and well, free of disease 2–10 yr. after treatment," refers to cases in the 1954–1963 group.

Diagnostic error on physical examination was impressive in the cases in which radical mastectomy was performed. For the decade, of 107 patients judged to be in Class A clinically, 38 per cent had nodes involved pathologically, and in 19 per cent this involvement was extensive. Conversely, of 48 patients judged to be in clinical Class B, palpable nodes were not involved with cancer in almost half. These data accent the absolute necessity of obtaining a full axillary dissection specimen if one is to assess the extent of nodal involvement; it suggests that operative palpation will likewise have a high rate of diagnostic error.

The pathologic appearance of the tumors was of prognostic significance only at the two ends of the activity spectrum (Table 2), with the undifferentiated tumors and intraductal tumors showing strongly significant differences. The location of the lesion was likewise of little meaning except for the two most contrasting sites: the upper outer quadrant yielded 63 survivors out of 114 cases, or 55 per cent at two to ten years, whereas the inner and central groups had analogous figures at 32 out of 79, or 41 per cent. This difference is of only borderline significance, with chance-probability values between 0.1 and 0.05.

Postoperative irradiation was used after radical mastectomy in 64 patients, 50 of whom had nodal involvement (Table 3). The survival data at two to ten years show suggestive benefit only when the analysis is confined to those with heavily involved nodes. In this group 17 out of 35, or 49 per cent, survived with irradiation, and only 4 out of 10, or 40 per cent, without irradiation. In no subgroups were the differences any more marked than this, and in those without any nodes, and considering the five-year survivals only, there is a

TABLE 2. *PBBH Primaries — Results by Pathologic Types*

Group		Number of Cases
Total cases — 1954–1963		248
Died other causes or nonclassifiable	47	
Classifiable, at risk	201	
"Poorly differentiated adenocarcinoma," at risk		93
2–10 yr. alive and well	51/93(55%)(a)	
"Well-differentiated adenocarcinoma," at risk		81
2–10 yr. alive and well	41/81(51%)(b)	
"Undifferentiated tumors," at risk		10
2–10 yr. alive and well	1/10(10%)(c)	
"Intraductal tumors," at risk		17
2–10 yr. alive and well	15/17(88%)(d)	
Statistical significance* (a) versus (b)	= 0.5+	
Statistical significance (a) versus (c)	= 0.001−	
Statistical significance (a) + (b) versus (c)	= 0.001−	
Statistical significance (a) + (b) + (c) versus (d)	= 0.001−	

* Statistical significance, indicated for comparison in these tables, calculated by standard statistical methods based on pq product and critical ratio. Designation 0.5+ indicates that probability is 50% or greater that difference is due to chance alone, and significance level is nil; designation 0.001− signifies that the probability that differences are due to chance alone are <1:1000, and statistical significance is "highly significant." In between these extremes, designation such as 0.1/0.01 signifies probability that these differences are due to chance factors alone lies between 1:10 and 1:100 — a level considered "significant." In general, any chance-probability value <0.01 is considered "significant."

TABLE 3. *PBBH Primaries — Postoperative Irradiation*

	Radical Mastectomy Alone		Radical Mastectomy Plus Irradiation	
	Number	2–10 Yr. Alive and Well	Number	2–10 Yr. Alive and Well
No nodes	80	54 (68%)	14	8 (57%)
1 or minimal nodes	12	9 (75%)	15	10 (67%)
30%–50% nodes positive	10	4 (40%)	35	17 (49%)

None of the differences are significant (p > 0.4)

TABLE 4. *Early Oophorectomy in PBBH Primary Cases*

Group	Number of Cases		
Radical mastectomy, with no lymph nodes in specimen, at risk			54
Early oophorectomy		7/54(13%)	
2–10 yr. alive and well	4/7(57%)(a)		
No oophorectomy		47/54(87%)	
2–10 yr. alive and well	23/47(49%)(b)		
Statistical significance (a) versus (b) = 0.5+			
Radical mastectomy, with lymph nodes in specimen, at risk			122
Early oophorectomy		37/122(30%)	
2–10 yr. alive and well	12/37(32%)(c)		
No oophorectomy		85/122(70%)	
2–10 yr. alive and well	21/85(25%)(d)		
Statistical significance (c) versus (d) = 0.5/0.4			
Radical mastectomy all lymph-node groups, at risk			176
Early oophorectomy		44/176(25%)	
2–10 yr. alive and well	16/44(36%)(e)		
No oophorectomy		132/176(75%)	
2–10 yr. alive and well	44/132(34%)(f)		
Statistical significance (e) versus (f) = 0.5+			

slight bias in favor of the group receiving no irradiation. Supervoltage, high-dose irradiation, of the type most apt to be effective against lymph-node metastases was not available until the last year of this decade, and therefore is not evident in these statistics.

Examination of the menopausal status at the time of the treatment of primary disease showed that the best results were obtained in women who were treated before or precisely during the menopause. The more successful palliative treatment of secondary disease noted in patients whose primary tumors had been removed before the menopause might be traceable to the greater endocrine impact of early oophorectomy. Table 4 shows the data on early oophorectomy for the decade; there are no significant differences among groups. Patients referred here for treatment of secondary disease were a younger group than those with locally arising primary tumors. In the entire primary group, only 44, or 18 per cent, of the 248 had onset under the age of forty years whereas of those referred for treatment of secondary disease the onset was under forty-five in 87, or 39 per cent, of 221. This tendency to select youthful women for referral treatment of secondary disease is noteworthy. It probably reflects the concern of the referring physician for possible salvage of a younger woman with very ominous prognostic developments, rather than any intrinsic biologic property of the tumor. It also has the statistical effect of loading the data on secondary disease with comparatively youthful women who had primary lesions.

4

FOLLOW-UP DATA: THE FREE INTERVAL, RECURRENCE AND METASTASES

AFTER the primary treatment, the patient enters an interval free of overt disease. In approximately one-half of all patients treated for cancer of the breast, this interval will last for the rest of her life. Whatever its duration, the patient has several problems to face: cosmetic factors, radiation, surgical menopause, the opposite breast, and follow-up examination for recurrence.

As for the *opposite breast*, figures for recurrence range from 7 to 12 per cent, always with some lingering confusion over whether the second breast is involved by metastases or new primary disease. Among the Brigham patients, 180 were alive and well three or more years after primary treatment, and in these patients the opposite breast became involved in 22, or 12.2 per cent. Three of the 22 had secondary operations on the opposite breast usually for removal before radiotherapy. These bilateral involvements were considered to be a "second primary" tumor in most cases.

Should patients have a "prophylactic" simple mastectomy on the uninvolved side if they have survived for three years or more after radical mastectomy? Certainly, a strong case can be made out for such a course, especially if palpable lumps are present, chronic cystic mastitis is found, or the breast is large and pendulous.

If the patient has a strong family history of breast cancer, removal of the contralateral breast becomes an even more pressing matter.

Mammography has been helpful in examination of the breast in high-risk situations. The reports by Egan,[58] Gershon-Cohen et al.,[59] Witten and Thurber[60] and Byrne and his associates[61] should be consulted. Byrne et al.[61] have explored the use of mammography in a study of the opposite breast after mastectomy. They found 6 cases in 102 patients followed for several years; in 1 case, the tumor was discovered eighty-four months after the initial mastectomy. They recommended the examination be carried out at six-month intervals. The dose to the skin ranged around 6 to 8 rads, with a probable depth dose of around 2 to 3 rads.

Study of the patient's family should be carried out during this interval, with particular emphasis on sisters and aunts and the patient's mother if she is still living. If the patient has daughters, a time should be chosen when they are of an appropriate age to discuss the possible risk they run and steps that might be taken to minimize it over the coming years.

Procedures for follow-up observation must strike a reasonable balance between overzealous examination and neglect. Repeated x-ray study may reveal metastases at the earliest possible moment, but it arouses the patient's apprehensions anew each time it is undertaken. Follow-up examination every three months for three years and every six months for the next three years seems to be acceptable.* No matter how cautious the routine, one is distressed at the frequency with which

---

* An informed patient, aware of her general problem but not depressed by overemphasis on detailed prognosis, is most likely to accept careful follow-up study and further steps in treatment as needed.

TABLE 5. *Length of Free Interval and Overall Survival or Response to Palliation in PBBH Primary and All Secondary Cases*

Group		Number of Cases	
PBBH primary cases, 1954–1963			248
Developed secondary disease (1954–1963)		110/248(44%)	
Clinical Class D when first seen			29
Clinical Classes A, B and C, at risk			219
Developed secondary disease		81/219 (37%)	
Free interval evaluated			81
Free interval < 1 yr.		23/81(28%)	
2–10 yr. alive and well	None		
Free interval 1-5 yr.		43/81(53%)	
2–10 yr. alive and well	6/43(14%)(a)		
Free interval > 5 yr.		15/81(19%)	
2–10 yr. alive and well	2/15(13%)(b)		
Statistical significance (a) versus (b) = 0.5+			
Referred secondary cases			213
Clinical Class D when first treated			9
Free interval evaluated			204
Free interval < 1 yr.		72/204(35%)	
2–10 yr. alive and well	3/72(4%)		
Free interval 1-5 yr.		101/204(50%)	
2–10 yr. alive and well	12/101(12%)		
Free interval > 5 yr.		31/204(15%)	
2–10 yr. alive and well	4/31(13%)		
All secondary cases treated with known free intervals			285
Free interval < 2 yr.		163/285(57%)	
Positive response to therapy	88/163(54%)(c)		
Free interval > 2 yr.		122/285(43%)	
Positive response to therapy	85/122(70%)(d)		
Statistical significance (c) versus (d) = 0.01/0.005			

the first overt evidences of disease arise in the interval between two examinations, and in retrospect appear to have been minimally present on at least one previous examination.

The emotional stress of repeated follow-up examinations is greatly heightened if a renewed surgical attack on the breast or axilla will become a byproduct of any positive finding. For this reason, as well as many others, one can scarcely embrace the concept of delayed axillary dissection.

The patient's free interval comes to an end when recurrence or metastases are found. The duration of the free interval and the precise location of the first metastases are of primary and controlling importance in the expectation of response to subsequent therapy. It is in the slowly growing tumors that endocrine palliation is most effective, and a free interval of more than twenty-four months is most favorable. The data on the free interval and first metastases both in the PBBH primary cases and in the referred secondary cases are presented in Tables 5 and 6. As shown in Table 5, both survival and response data clearly favor the longer free intervals.

The prognostic significance of a positive response to palliative therapy, as based on the anatomy of the first metastasis, is indicated in Table 6. Analysis of these cases shows that there is little correlation between the length of the free interval and the anatomy of the first metastasis. These two prognostic factors, therefore, become additive in significance — for example, if a patient has a long free interval, with a first recurrence in local skin or in bone, the likelihood of a positive response* to palliative therapy rises to 70 per cent or higher.

---

* The term "positive response" as used here includes both subjec-

TABLE 6. *First Metastasis and Overall Palliative Success
in Patients with Secondary Disease*

Group		Number of Cases
All secondary disease		323
All cases — positive response		
to subsequent therapy		192/323(59%)
First metastases and response rates		
Bone		111/323(34%)
Positive response	70/111(63%)	
Skin, local (67 cases)		
or elsewhere (6 cases)		73/323(21%)
Positive response	46/72(63%)	
Ipsilateral lymph node		50/323(16%)
Positive response	33/50(66%)	
Lungs or pleura		50/323(15%)
Positive response	25/50(50%)	
Viscera, brain or other		28/323(9%)
Positive response	12/28(43%)	

Establishment of Base-Line Indexes of Growth and Regression

Before anything is done for the treatment of what is
assumed to be a recurrence of cancer of the breast, every
effort must be made to establish that the disease is actually present and to discern the degree to which it is
progressive. Diagnosis is not always a simple matter.
When the disease spreads to lungs, brain and bone,
meddlesome biopsy must take a position subsidiary to
clinical likelihood and radiologic appearances. In any
large series there will be many patients in whom extensive therapy for metastatic breast cancer must be undertaken without any positive histologic proof of the
presence of the disease.

---

tive and objective relief, and has a higher incidence than objective
remission.

Many diagnostic procedures also establish indexes that will later be useful in establishing the rate of growth of the metastases or regression in response to palliative treatment. These include measurements and records of the size of the lesions, hematologic profile, serum calcium and phosphorus concentration, lactic dehydrogenase and serum transaminase and, in cases in which the skeleton is involved, twenty-four-hour determinations of urinary calcium.

If only one or two small nests of disease are present but scarcely active and virtually asymptomatic, in any site, the simplest possible treatment should be advised. This is usually local irradiation. Further developments can be awaited before one moves on to more drastic measures. If this isolated recurrence takes the form of a small subcutaneous nodule with freely movable full thickness of skin over it on the chest wall, local total excision with a generous margin of normal tissue and local irradiation will often be followed by survival for many years. These *subcutaneous* metastases are in a sharp contrast to *intracutaneous* spread, which is very destructive, difficult to control and causes severe symptoms. Donegan et al.,[62] who have carried out a biostatistical study of locally recurrent breast disease, advise an aggressive attack on small local recurrences because of this possibility.

Unfortunately, recurrent disease is usually quite progressive, as indicated both by symptoms or film sequences and by chemical indexes, and it is usually quite characteristic in its appearance. Patient and surgeon are then faced with a certain prospect: they are beginning a course that will last for one month to ten or more years and, although the patient need hardly be apprised of the fact, the course will certainly terminate fatally.

Oophorectomy

About 50 per cent of patients who are within ten years of the menopause may be expected to respond favorably to a therapeutic oophorectomy undertaken to palliate symptomatic metastatic breast cancer.[52] This favorable response rate continues for some years, gradually falling to a lower level by the age of sixty-five or seventy.

Many patients found to have recurrent or metastatic disease will state that an oophorectomy has been carried out years before, and in some cases irradiation castration will be claimed as part of the treatment of the primary disease, or as a prior therapy for some such disease as uterine fibroids. In either case, the surgeon should make certain that ovarian estrogen production has been completely wiped out before he proceeds to some other and less certain form of palliative therapy. The vaginal smear or urinary sedimentary cytology is useful here, and this may be their chief utility in the treatment of this disease. In the vaginal smear, cornification figures higher than 15 per cent are due to the presence of ovarian estrogens and are virtually never due to adrenal estrogens alone.

If the patient has not previously had an oophorectomy, or if residual ovarian tissue appears to be present, oophorectomy should be carried out as the first step in treatment of recurrent or metastatic disease in any patient under the age of seventy-five. In some patients with very slowly advancing disease, a long free interval and no immediate threat to critical viscera, the solo therapeutic oophorectomy can be done, time being taken to observe the response to oophorectomy by as many measurable indexes as have been established by the baseline measurements. In patients with rapidly growing widespread or visceral disease, oophorectomy should be combined with adrenalectomy either at the same operation or within a few days. If the patient has disease that is so extensive as to make oophorectomy or adrenalectomy prohibitively dangerous, and yet the expectancy of life is reasonably good (a rare combination), castration can be done by irradiation. If this is undertaken, sufficient irradiation must be given to achieve the endocrine effects of oophorectomy, and this end point should be established by an appropriate change in vaginal cytology.

The concept of hyperplasia of cortical stroma[63] served notice that postmenopausal ovaries could still be potent sources of estrogen. This has been amply confirmed by many other data from estrogen analyses in the urine[64-66] and from cytologic studies of the vaginal or urinary sediment.[67] It remains uncertain exactly what fraction of patients who show significant estrogen production after the menopause actually have stromal hyperplasia.

5

PREDICTORS OF PALLIATIVE RESPONSE TO ADRENALECTOMY OR HYPOPHYSECTOMY

Clinical Predictors

MANY workers have sought some guide or sign by which the response to adrenalectomy or hypophysectomy might be predicted; these guides, predictors, indicators or discriminants can be divided into clinical and biochemical types.

Among the *clinical predictors,* the length of the free interval and the site of the first metastases predominate as by far the most significant. These have already been mentioned, and will not be dealt with further here.

The *age of the patient* is immaterial if either the free interval or the metastatic pattern is conclusive. Kleinfeld et al.[68] suggest that youthful patients with cancer of the breast have a very poor prognosis. This applies to very young patients — many in their twenties and thirties — a group in which the poor prognosis is demonstrated by a short free interval and ominous metastatic patterns.

Patients who are close to the *menopause* in our series have done as well as or slightly better than postmenopausal patients. The report of Smithers et al.[69] represents one of the few papers in the literature that would

43

agree with this conclusion about menopausal status; Smithers found that if the menopause follows closely the onset of breast cancer, the survival rate improves.

Predictors Based on Estrogen Secretion or Excretion

Despite the lack of any conclusive evidence that a decrease in body estrogens is the sole or even the chief cause of a favorable response to surgical manipulation of the endocrine glands, this hypothesis provided the basis for the first attempts to define with precision the endocrine status most favorable for palliative success.

There are abundant data indicating that after the normal menopause or surgical oophorectomy the level of estrogens in the blood and urine does not fall to zero, but instead may follow a slowly rising course after an initial fall, later falling to zero over the course of several decades. The data of Smith and Emerson[70] and of Nissen-Meyer and Sanner[64-66] are particularly significant in this connection. In 1963 Nissen-Meyer and Sanner[64] showed a slow decrease in the excretion of estrone and pregnanediol after the menopause, followed by a secondary rise with a new maximum about ten to fifteen years after the menopause. In a companion study the same investigators reported that removal of the ovaries lowered but did not eliminate the excretion of estrone after the age of forty-five.[65] The principal effect of oophorectomy was to remove the delayed peak occurring at fifty to fifty-five years of age. When corticosteroids were added to the treatment, however, estrogen and pregnanediol excretion both were reduced to essentially zero. The authors found that ovarian irradiation (2400 R over a six-day period) was as effective as oophorectomy in reducing the estrogen level. It should be noted that this dose is almost six times that used by Paterson and Russell[54] in their negative study of x-ray castration.

Response to Prior Therapeutic Oophorectomy

Long considered the best indicator of subsequent responsiveness to adrenalectomy or hypophysectomy, the prior oophorectomy response is rarely available as a criterion, and is not a very reliable one. Table 7 shows the remarkable variety of prior pelvic surgery carried out in the 323 patients treated for secondary disease. Of 140 oophorectomies, only 40 were performed in the absence of significant additional therapy that would cloud the interpretation, and in only 30 was the operation done in a situation in which the "objective remission" could accurately be gauged by measurable changes. Thus, in only 9 per cent of all the patients treated for secondary disease was prior oophorectomy available as a criterion; of the 131 patients in this group who later had adrenalectomy or hypophysectomy, in 19, or 15 per cent, a prior therapeutic oophorectomy was carried out in a setting that would permit its use as a criterion for subsequent palliation.

Turning from the availability of the response to oophorectomy, one finds conflicting evidence of its reliability as a criterion of the likelihood of further palliative success. A recent study by Fracchia et al.[71] states that of 124 patients who had a prior favorable response to oophorectomy, 46, or 38 per cent, had a remission after adrenalectomy, whereas of the 36 patients who failed to respond to oophorectomy, only 7 had a favorable response to adrenalectomy. Data from the PBBH experience on the reliability of the oophorectomy criterion are shown in Table 8. In only half the cases was

TABLE 7. *Prior Oophorectomy as a Criterion in Patients with Secondary Disease:* Availability

Group		Number of Cases
PBBH primary cases (females)		248
Prior oophorectomy		20/248(8%)
Prior hysterectomy or unilateral oophorectomy		22/248(9%)
Prior hysterectomy and bilateral oophorectomy		42/248(17%)
Referred secondaries		213
Prior oophorectomy		13/213(6%)
Prior hysterectomy or unilateral oophorectomy		14/213(7%)
Total prior genitectomy		27/213(13%)
Total secondaries		323
Early oophorectomy (within 1 mo. of mastectomy)		87/323(26%)
Solo therapeutic oophorectomy		40/323(12%)
Combined therapeutic oophorectomy		100/323(31%)
With hypophysectomy	4/100	
With adrenalectomy	12/100	
With hormone therapy	48/100	
With radiation or other	36/100	
Fraction of therapeutic oophorectomies done solo		40/140(29%)
Solo therapeutic oophorectomy done in measurable response setting		30/323(9%)
Total secondary cases later treated by adrenalectomy or hypophysectomy (1954–1963)		131
Solo therapeutic oophorectomy done in measurable response setting, in patients later having adrenalectomy or hypophysectomy		19/131(15%)

the subsequent palliative response (to adrenalectomy or hypophysectomy) consistent with the oophorectomy response.

Biochemical Discriminants

From 1960 on a group of authors in London[72-75] began to report a series of studies based initially on a retrospective analysis of urinary hormone excretion in pa-

TABLE 8. *Prior Oophorectomy as a Criterion in Patients with Secondary Disease: Reliability*

Group	Number of Cases
Adrenalectomy (54 cases) and hypophysectomy (77 cases), 1954–1963	131
Prior therapeutic oophorectomy of any type*	82/131(63%)
Criterion-acceptable oophorectomy	19/82(23%)
Response-consistent†	9/19(47%)

* Of these 82 prior therapeutic oophorectomies, 33 were done in adrenalectomy cases and 49 in hypophysectomy cases.

† Of these 9 cases in which response to adrenalectomy or hypophysectomy was consistent with prior oophorectomy, patients were about equally divided between those who obtained favorable response to both and those who did not.

tients undergoing hypophysectomy and adrenalectomy. These data were then correlated with the palliative result achieved.

At about the same time, data from this hospital began to accumulate, demonstrating that inhibition of adrenal function by the administration of corticosteroids was associated with an excellent palliative response in some cases. By operative and postmortem study of adrenal histology[76] it was shown that corticosteroid treatment produced functional inhibition of the adrenal glands and a parallel anatomic atrophy. Studies were therefore undertaken to contrast the maximum secretory capacity of the gland under ACTH stimulation with the size and histology of the adrenal gland and with the palliative result achieved by its removal.

The Bulbrook–Hayward Discriminant

To carry out this study the patient is placed on baseline urine steroid collections to measure the daily excretion of 17-hydroxycorticosteroids and etiocholanolone. From these data a discriminant is calculated as follows:

$$D = 80 - 80 \, (17\text{-OH}) + (\text{Etio}),$$

where:

        D = discriminant function

 17-OH = twenty-four-hour urinary excretion of 17-hydroxycorticosteroids in milligrams

   Etio = twenty-four-hour urinary excretion of etiocholanolone in micrograms.

It is noted that the value for D (the discriminant) becomes strongly positive when the etiocholanolone figure is high in relation to the 17-hydroxycorticosteroid. This discriminant value varies from about −750 to +2000, and the more strongly positive results are correlated with palliative success.

As an example of the type of data presented, the

British authors found that, including all ages and menopausal groups, those with a positive value for D among a group of 70 cases had a 39 per cent palliative success rate for adrenalectomy and hypophysectomy. Those with a negative value for D had only an 8 per cent success rate among 64 patients. This difference is strongly significant. When to these numbers information on the free interval was added, improvement in prediction of success was not notable, but prediction of failure became virtually absolute.

Biochemical discriminants should be used with great caution to deny adrenalectomy to patients if the free interval is long or if certain other clinical data (such as metastatic pattern and age at menopause) are favorable. If, on the other hand, the clinical discriminants are unfavorable and the biochemical discriminant is likewise negative, one can assure the patient and her family that the palliative operation is not to be undertaken and that medicinal therapy of some sort should be substituted for it.

The Incremental-Ratio Discriminant

Research in the Surgical Laboratories of the Peter Bent Brigham Hospital has been devoted to a study of adrenal structure (size, cortical thickness and nuclear cell counts) and functions (with ACTH tests) in relation to the palliation achieved by their removal. Function has been measured during ACTH stimulation, a procedure based on the conviction that the maximum secretion evoked by stimulation should be more representative of adrenal capacity than the resting values alone. Two days of resting secretion are contrasted with two days under stimulation. The increment in secretory activity, measured by urinary excretion and evoked by

ACTH, is then expressed as a fraction of the resting value (incremental ratio). All collections are carried out in the hospital; creatinine excretion is measured throughout, and all values are corrected to the simultaneous creatinine. The urine 17-hydroxycorticosteroids and total urinary 17-ketosteroids are measured and expressed in milligrams per gram of creatinine. The results of these studies are currently being reported and summarized;[77] a D value is calculated from the endocrine data, as follows:

$$D = -4.5 + 0.44(\text{17-OH I.R.}) + 0.73(\text{17-K I.R.}) + 0.037 \text{ F.I.,}$$

where:
17-OH I.R. = incremental ratio for urinary 17-hydroxycorticosteroid excretion, corrected for creatinine, and based on forty-eight hours resting and forty-eight hours stimulated (40 units of ACTH given intravenously per day over six to eight hours)
17-K I.R. = same for total urinary 17-ketosteroids
F.I. = free interval in months

When the value for D is positive, correlation is with a favorable response, and when it is negative, with palliative failure.* As an example of the ability of this discriminant, it correctly identified 12 out of 15, or 80 per cent, of the responders in one series, and 12 out of 16, or 75 per cent, of the nonresponders. It should be emphasized that this study, like the initial report of Bulbrook et al.,[72] is a retrospective one. The discriminant has yet to be put to the test of case selection, and even then it may have great difficulty competing with the use of the free interval and first metastatic sites.

* We are indebted to Dr. Anthony F. Bartholomay and the Biomathematics Division for extensive collaboration throughout this study, particularly in the analysis of correlations and regression equations for urinary hormone excretion and adrenal size and for the identification of the most effective discriminant function.

6

ADRENALECTOMY AND HYPOPHYSECTOMY

Acceptability of Surgical Palliation — Overall Success Rate

ALTHOUGH the fractional incidence of palliative success appears to be about the same for hormone therapy and an unselected series of adrenalectomies or hypophysectomies, it has been a virtually universal experience, and certainly that of our group, that the operations provide a longer and more complete respite from the disease than do the hormones in the patients who do respond favorably.

Even though the response to palliative treatment can be graded according to objective remissions, these criteria are not the only ones that affect the value judgments of patient and doctor. Many patients have disease that is highly symptomatic but is not easily visible or measurable, and they experience subjective relief that is so profound as to demand inclusion in the affirmative column. On the negative side, mere failure to achieve an objective remission is not a sufficient indictment: in some patients the treatment appears to be a total waste of time and effort, and in some patients the disease quite evidently progresses at an increased rate after treatment, both medical and surgical.[78] For these reasons, in the tables that follow, "positive result" indicates a signifi-

51

TABLE 9. *Overall Palliative Success in Secondary Disease*

Group	Number of Cases
Total with secondary disease	323
PBBH primary cases	110
Referred secondary cases	213
Positive response (all modalities)	192/323(59%)
Objective and subjective	135/323(42%)
Objective only	5/323(2%)
Subjective only	52/323(16%)
Negative response (all modalities)	88/323(27%)
No clear benefit	64/323(20%)
Waste of time and effort	24/323(7%)
Indeterminate result (all modalities)	43/323(13%)
Too short to evaluate	15/323(5%)
Inconclusive	28/323(9%)
Positive response in treatment of secondary disease in PBBH primary cases	38/110(35%)(a)
Positive response in treatment of referred secondary cases	135/213(63%)(b)
Statistical significance (a) versus (b) < 0.001	

cant combination of subjective and objective improvement, and "negative result" includes both patients who had no clear benefit and those in whom the entire effort was deemed a waste of time.

In all, 323 patients were seen and studied for treatment of secondary and metastatic disease that followed a primary treatment modality, usually radical mastectomy. The overall success rates are shown in Table 9. The positive response rate varies from 35 to 63 per cent, being highest in referred secondary cases, a group preselected from referring physicians. This success rate seems high as compared with the literature of a few year ago; yet one must recall that it reflects increasing experience in the selection of patients and increasing use of therapeutic combinations most apt to yield success, as based on the earlier data.

At the other end of the scale, the results were judged to be entirely negative in 27 per cent of the cases. Among these negative results are included only 12 of the 24 patients who showed a clear exacerbation on androgens and estrogens (as discussed below) because, although these exacerbations were often severe, the patients later obtained good results from other palliative steps.

Surgical Hypophysectomy

First carried out about fifteen years ago, and now reported from several centers,[79,80] surgical hypophysectomy remains an effective method for achieving palliation in advanced carcinoma of the breast, and should theoretically be more effective than adrenalectomy. This theoretical advantage is traceable to the fact that the operation removes not only the source of the adrenocorticotrophic hormones but also a hormone or hormones that appear to stimulate the breast directly. There is now sufficient information from our experience and from the literature to indicate clearly that despite this theoretical advantage, hypophysectomy achieves no improvement in palliative success rate over adrenalectomy, and that the remissions, when they occur, are of no greater duration.[81]

By 1960 it was evident that hypophysectomy had three important contrasts with adrenalectomy when carried out by the same surgical staff in the same hospital and with the same patient population.[82-84] In the first place, surgical hypophysectomy is a somewhat more difficult, protracted and challenging technical procedure than adrenalectomy. Secondly, the course after hypophysectomy is more difficult to manage, and complications when they do occur are much more severe since they are apt to involve the cranial cavity or the brain itself. Thirdly, hormone replacement is considerably more complicated after hypophysectomy because of the small but persistent incidence of diabetes insipidus. For these reasons, the overall hospital mortality and morbidity are significantly greater for hypophysectomy than for adrenalectomy. There may be some occasions, however, in which hypophysectomy remains the preferred operation, such as the association of breast cancer with pregnancy.

Table 10 summarizes the hypophysectomies and adrenalectomies carried out at this hospital. Some of these cases have previously been reported,[80] but the follow-up information has not previously been indicated. Hospital mortality and morbidity are higher in hypophysectomy, and objective remission rates are not significantly different; the table fails to emphasize the

TABLE 10. *Summary of Results of Hypophysectomy and Adrenalectomy in Secondary Disease*

Operation	Number of Cases	Hospital Deaths	Complications	Cases of Diabetes Insipidus	Objective Remissions	Statistical Significance a vs. b
Hypophysectomy (1954–62)	77*	7/77(9.1%)	24/77(31%)	37/77(48%)†	31/77(40%)(a)	0.5+
Adrenalectomy (1961–65)	86‡	3/86(4.0%)	3/86(4%)	0	44/86(51%)(b)	

* Fifty-three of these 77 hypophysectomies previously reported.[80]
† Refers to all cases requiring vasopressin; only 8 of these patients had severe continuing difficulty with this complication.
‡ Additional 8 patients undergoing adrenalectomy, not included here. Six operated on very early in our experience and before start of this series: of these, 1 clearly made worse by operation, as previously reported.[78] Two additional patients seen in consulation here and operated upon elsewhere.

many patients (about 70 per cent) who went through hypophysectomy smoothly, had only transient diabetes insipidus and achieved fine palliation. The hypophysectomies were carried out in the years before 1962; the greater experience in case selection was therefore not available as it was for the more recent adrenalectomy group. The higher mortality in some part reflects this because several of the deaths after hypophysectomy were due to the excessively advanced or preterminal stage of the disease at the time of operation.

The large series of hypophysectomies being reported by Ray[79] presents a number of contrasting features. There were 630 cases treated by hypophysectomy between 1952 and 1966. The mortality was 7.3 per cent in the first 218 cases but later fell to 2.0 per cent. Visual-field defects were encountered only rarely; about 30 per cent of patients lost their sense of smell, and diabetes insipidus was a continuing problem in about 20 per cent of cases. The palliative success rate was approximately 42 per cent for the whole series, with some individual variations among groups. No attempt was made to evaluate the completeness of the operation either by cortisone withdrawal or by evocative tests of ACTH production. There is no other report of such a large and successful series of surgical hypophysectomies in the American literature.

If hypophysectomy could be carried out in some way that completely avoided cerebral or neurologic complications, the question of completeness would still remain. There is increasing evidence[85] that most hypophysectomies performed in this country and Great Britain have been subtotal. The detailed endocrinologic study required for such a conclusion has generally not been carried out in the larger reported series.

Yttrium Hypophysectomy

Yttrium hypophysectomy has been developed in part to meet the need for a simple method of pituitary removal that would not carry the hazard of a full-dress craniotomy, and might even lend itself to very short-term hospitalization. Among others who have pioneered this procedure, special mention should be made of Forrest.[86-88] In his most recent publication[87] he makes it clear that the screw-implant yttrium hypophysectomy is still in an experimental phase. He states that it is "less reliable than adrenalectomy" but points out its simplicity and the fact that the period of hospitalization is only four or five days. The occurrence of fatal meningitis in 2 per cent of cases, extraocular palsy in 2 per cent, rhinorrhea in 3 per cent and visual impairment in about 1.5 per cent, with a mortality of 3.0 to 4.4 per cent, indicates the absolute minimums for these morbidity components obtainable in the hands of experts.

A special application for yttrium hypophysectomy might be found in the treatment of exacerbations occurring after a favorable adrenalectomy response. Forrest[88] reports that in a substantial series of patients he made this attempt and that the result was negative.

Adrenalectomy

The simultaneous bilateral posterior twelfth-rib approach enables one to carry out a total adrenalectomy expeditiously and with low morbidity and mortality. The operation is technically challenging only when the adrenal gland and the vena cava are contiguously invaded by tumor. The experience in this hospital has not produced the complications reported by some, such as trauma to the tail of the pancreas or the hollow viscera; nonetheless, particular care must be taken to dissect the adrenal glands completely and to identify and ligate the adrenal vein under direct vision bilaterally.

The postoperative course has shown itself to be smooth, with early ambulation and a prompt return to normal diet. Replacement therapy is simple: hydrocortisone, at the rate of 300 mg. per day, is administered intravenously for two or three days, followed by a reduction to a daily maintenance dose of 50 to 75 mg. given by mouth. Alpha-fluorohydrocortisone is given in the amount of 0.1 mg. every other day. The patient is usually ready to go home by the seventh day, unless chemotherapy is being begun, and in such cases, a few extra days in the hospital are well justified.

The results shown in Table 10 summarize the data on our first 86 adrenalectomies performed since 1961. As noted, the mortality for adrenalectomy is low (4 per cent). Two of the postoperative deaths were traceable to the selection of patients who had crippling and threatening visceral involvement; none could be ascribed to such complications as hemorrhage, infection or pulmonary embolism unrelated to the cancer itself. Several of the patients showing objective remissions had breast cancer involving threatening visceral areas, particularly the lungs; such stray results always constitute a temptation to operate on patients with late disease.

A sampling of published series of adrenalectomies[71,81,89-103] shows that only 8[71,81,89,91-93,101,103] reported more than 50 cases; the total compilation includes 1895 cases. In the larger groups the hospital mortality ranged from 4.5 to 16 per cent, and the response rate, defined according to a variety of criteria, from 28 to 45 per cent.

In general, the patients with no response may be expected to live for about six months, and those with a response for eighteen to twenty-four months.

It is noteworthy that each successive year of our experience with adrenalectomy has seen an improvement in the response rate. It would be satisfying to ascribe the increasing success of adrenalectomy at this hospital to some external factor such as the use of biochemical discriminants or the concomitant use of chemotherapy (discussed below). Neither of these can be used to explain the steadily improved results, which appear to be due to the increasing experience in selection of cases, and particularly in avoidance of operations on patients in whom the outlook for palliative success is dim.

The medicinal use of corticosteroids for palliative medication produces marked adrenal atrophy; an unsettled question in such cases bears on the palliative response as a predictor of subsequent adrenalectomy response when the corticosteroids ultimately fail. The adrenal atrophy resulting from corticosteroids is maximal after about six weeks; in animals[104] the addition of desoxycorticosterone or aldosterone does not produce any additional adrenal atrophy. When exacerbation occurs, the question arises whether the prior favorable response to corticosteroids indicates a responsive tumor that will respond later to adrenalectomy or whether the inhibition and atrophy produced by corticosteroid therapy render the adrenal gland so inconsequential that its subsequent removal accomplishes nothing for the patient. Our data suggest, but do not prove, that the removal of a markedly atrophic adrenal gland is less likely to achieve a palliative response than the removal of a previously untreated gland. For this reason we have avoided prolonged high-dose corticosteroid

TABLE 11. *Secondary Disease Adrenalectomy — Objective Remission Rate
in Relation to Grouping of Selection Factors*

Total adrenalectomies — 1961–1965	86
Free interval over 1 year	65/86(76%)
Objective remissions in patients with free interval over 1 year	39/65(60%)
Early hospital deaths or deaths from other causes	4
Free interval over 1 year, at risk, for palliative response	61
Objective remissions	39/61(64%)
Free interval over 1 year, treated also with 5-fluorouracil	10
Objective remissions	9/10(90%)

Note: Since the data analysis presented in Table 11 above, further experience with the combination of adrenalectomy and 5-fluorouracil shows an over-all objective remission rate of 31/47(66%); in those with free intervals of over 1 year, the rate was 19/24(79%). Those with free intervals of less than one year had a remission rate of 12/23(52%).

therapy in patients who are suitable for adrenalectomy.

Lastly, in relation to adrenalectomy should be mentioned the combined use of adrenalectomy with chemotherapy, consisting of 5-fluorouracil. In 1963 a cautious trial using 5-fluorouracil in high dose, starting on the third postoperative day after adrenalectomy, was begun. The chemotherapy did not complicate or add any hazard to the postoperative cortisone replacement.[105] Unexpected remissions were observed in several cases. According to this procedure 5-fluorouracil is begun at high dosage by intravenous infusion on or about the third postoperative day after adrenalectomy; after six days of this treatment, the drug is given at weekly intervals. Although experience is too small to offer any long-term evaluation, the combination of adrenalectomy and chemotherapy appears to provide an encouraging improvement over the results of adrenalectomy alone.

As shown in Table 11, an objective response rate of 64 per cent is obtained by adrenalectomy in patients with a free interval of greater than one year. It is of interest that no woman with a free interval of less than twelve months has responded to adrenalectomy alone, while the response rate for such patients receiving combined 5-fluorouracil therapy and adrenalectomy remains at 52 per cent.

7

MEDICINAL PALLIATION
(HORMONES AND CHEMOTHERAPY
AND LOCAL RADIOTHERAPY)

PATIENTS with metastatic disease who are judged unsuitable for adrenalectomy should receive hormone therapy. On the basis of our present experience the combination of cortisone by mouth with 5-fluorouracil intravenously yields the most satisfactory results. In the following sections these and other medicinal methods are briefly reviewed.

Estrogens and Androgens

The administration of estrogens demonstrated for the first time the medicinal palliation of advanced carcinoma of the breast,[1] just as Beatson's removal of the ovary had demonstrated the first surgical palliation. Despite the historic significance of estrogen administration the sex hormones have become less useful in this disease as other methods are explored. In addition, experience early in the activities of the tumor group of the Peter Bent Brigham Hospital[49,50] showed that most patients with cancer of the breast under sixty-five years of age demonstrated an increased growth of the disease under estrogen therapy. This is reminiscent of the urinary calcium cycle from the normal menstrual period

63

in patients with bone metastases reported by Pearson and his associates.[48] These drug-induced exacerbations naturally led to poor therapeutic results with estrogens, and several serious exacerbations — 2 deaths — have resulted from the administration of estrogens in our series. Hypercalcemia appears to be the most severe early complication of therapy, and one virtually confined to the sex hormone; the toxicity of estrogen treatment in carcinoma of the breast lies primarily in hypercalcemia. Jessiman et al.[106] reported 59 episodes of severe hypercalcemia in 33 patients out of a group of 145 treated at this hospital. Although hypercalcemia can be a spontaneous manifestation of rapid growth of advanced cancer of the breast, metastatic to the skeleton, a significant fraction of these cases could be directly traced to the therapeutic administration of estrogens or androgens. For these reasons one is loath to use the hormones in young women who are suitable for other forms of therapy: better clinical results, free of this hazard, are obtained with surgical adrenalectomy or the medicinal use of corticosteroids.

Hypercalcemia and, more rarely, hypocalcemia have now been reported by many workers.[20,107-110] Extensive discussion of this subject will be avoided here except to indicate that hypercalcemia can occur after androgen as well as after estrogen therapy, presumably by dint of biochemical interconversion. The complication has never been observed on cortisone therapy, and corticosteroids are a most important therapeutic measure for the treatment of hypercalcemia. The symptoms of hypercalcemia are manifold, and the complications can be lethal.

In very elderly patients, in whom the disease has established itself in an estrogen-free environment, the palliative results of estrogen continue to be remarkable, as initially reported by Nathanson and Kelley.[1] It is in these cases that the sex hormones continue to be most useful.

Most of the androgenic hormones that produce palliation in this disease also have severe side effects, such as facial hirsutism and changes in psyche and libido. Interconversion to estrogens appears to be as real clinically as it is biochemically; it has never been proved beyond question that androgens per se do not cause hypercalcemia. Nissen-Meyer and Sanner[64] have demonstrated interconversion by finding large increases in estrogen excretion in patients given testosterone. If testosterone is given at the rate of 500 mg. per week, interconversion of only 1 per cent will produce 5000 μg. of estrogen, an amount more than ten times the daily estrogen secretion of a menstruating young woman. Emerson and his associates[111] reported conversion of 17-ethyl-19-nortestosterone to estrogens, demonstrating that some of the modified testosterone and possibly hormones occupying an intermediate position between progesterone and testosterone are capable of conversion to estrogens. This type of conversion has been demonstrated by several other workers.[112-115]

Dao and Nemoto[116] report an interesting contrast of 261 patients studied at the Roswell Park Hospital in Buffalo, N.Y., of whom a third were treated with adrenalectomy, a third with fluoxymesterone and a third with other test androgens.* Forty-five per cent of

---

* Because of the possibility that minor changes in the androgen molecule confer some special benefit, a broad-scale national effort was devoted to the study of the clinical significance of minor config-

TABLE 12. *Sex Steroids — Estrogens and Androgens — in Secondary Disease*

Treatment		Number of Cases
Total secondary disease		323
Total courses androgens		154/323(48%)
Testosterone or related drugs	110	
Androstanopyrazole*	39	
Dromostanolone	5	
Positive response		49/154(32%)
Clear exacerbation (testosterone)		7/110(6%)
Estrogen stimulation tests		19/323(6%)
Exacerbation		16/19(84%)
Total courses estrogens		84/323(26%)
Total solo estrogen therapy > 60 days		34/84(40%)
Positive response	15/34(44%)	
Clear exacerbations	17/84(20%)	
Fatal exacerbations	2/17(12%)	

* Positive response rate for androstanopyrazole, 10/39(26%).

86 patients with adrenalectomy had an objective remission whereas only 16 per cent of those on fluoxymesterone had a response. The authors noted a significant loss of patients capable of undergoing adrenalectomy if hormones were used first.

Table 12 shows a summary of our experience with androgen and estrogen therapy. Positive response rates of approximately 30 to 40 per cent are not difficult to obtain, but the duration of these responses is relatively short (three to eight months). The number of clear exacerbation is impressive.

urational changes in the steroid molecule, largely in the androgens.[117] From none of these studies has any qualitative change arisen to indicate a new order of magnitude of therapeutic effectiveness. Differences have often been at the borderline statistical level, and it appears that the patients might have been better off if adrenalectomy had been carried out.

Progestins

A number of hormones chemically related to progesterone have been offered for the treatment of this disease. They have not appeared to offer any significant increase in beneficial result; marked hypercalcemia has been recorded in at least 1 of these,[20] and, as with estrogen and androgen in the middle-aged group, one can rightly question the use of these hormones, when adrenalectomy or corticosteroids can yield beneficial results without the hazardous side effect of hypercalcemia.

Corticosteroids

The administration of cortisone or its various synthetic analogues in low dosage has resulted in remarkable palliation in many patients with carcinoma of the breast. Although corticosteroid therapy is neither free of hazard nor unaccompanied by unpleasant side effects, it can be given without fear that the disease itself will be stimulated and exacerbated thereby. On this score alone, and wholly aside from other considerations, cortisone has achieved a much greater usefulness than either estrogens or androgens in our series of patients; its major action is presumably due to a decrease in the production of estrogens by the adrenal gland.[118]

When corticosteroid responses were first observed, it was considered that they might be nonspecific, psychologic or emotional. It was then observed that corticosteroids can sharply reduce the calcium excretion in patients with bone metastases and hypercalcuria.[119] In patients suffering from hypercalcemia, the administration of corticosteroids often lowers the serum calcium concentration while the urinary calcium excretion is also falling, indicating that total calcium mobilization from bone is being reduced.[106] This change is the more remarkable in view of the fact that the usual effect of corticosteroids on skeletal salt metabolism in older women is one of osteoporosis and increasing hypercalcuria. The disappearance of pulmonary metastases and the recalcification of skeletal metastases leave little doubt that corticosteroid administration affects the disease favorably as well as improving the patient's sense of well-being.

Corticosteroid remissions can last as long as a year. The usual duration is about six months; atypical metastatic patterns have been reported as a complication by Sherlock and Hartmann[120] and observed in our patients likewise. For these several reasons, corticosteroid therapy does not provide the same satisfaction for the patient as adrenalectomy; in addition, corticosteroid complications are sometimes quite bothersome.

These complications consist of exacerbation of latent diabetes, duodenal ulcer, hirsutism, rounding of the face and changing of the bodily contours. The changes appear to be reduced by the concomitant administration of large amounts of potassium. Remarkable degrees of weight gain are also a nuisance. It is of interest that patients given 50 to 75 mg. of cortisone a day after adrenalectomy give no evidence whatsoever of hyperadrenocorticism whereas in patients with normal adrenal glands in place who receive the same dose there will be severe evidence of hyperadrenocorticism. In 1 case death appeared to result from a combination of advanced disease and inability to take cortisone by mouth that was recognized only belatedly when corticosteroids were finally given parenterally without effect; adrenal insufficiency due to prolonged adrenal inhibition certainly played a part in this fatal outcome.

Table 13 presents data from the experience with corticosteroid therapy at the Peter Bent Brigham Hospital. The drug has been used very widely. Positive response rates run from 41 to 57 per cent, depending upon the series division, but major complications run as high as 31 per cent in patients who have received the

TABLE 13. *Summary of Corticosteroid Therapy in Secondary Disease*

Therapy	Number of Cases	
Total secondary disease		323
Total patients receiving		223/323(69%)
corticosteroids		
> 60 days, major or		
solo courses	79	
Positive response	45/79(57%)	
Major feature of		
multiple courses	111	
Positive response	45/111(41%)	
Total solo or		
major courses	190	
Positive response	90/190(47%)	
Minor courses	25	
Positive response	5/25(20%)	
Given to control		
postoperative		
exacerbation	8	
Positive response	4/8(50%)	
Total solo or		
major courses		190
Major complications of		
corticosteroids		59/190(31%)
Cushingoid features	32/190(17%)	
Weight gain	9/190(5%)	
Diabetes mellitus	7/190(4%)	
Bleeding duodenal ulcer	1/190(1%)	
Other*	10/190(5%)	
Clear exacerbation of		
disease	0/190(0%)	

* These 10 patients include 1 who evidently died of drug-induced adrenal insufficiency; after prolonged corticosteroid therapy, illness supervened; patient did not take her cortisone as instructed and later died of combination of advanced cancer with adrenal insufficiency.

drug for a long time. It should be noted that these complications, although referred to as "major," include such things as round face and weight gain — hardly a threat as compared with hypercalcemia in patients treated with sex hormones.

At present the greatest usefulness of corticosteroids appears to reside in their availability as an effective alternative to surgical adrenalectomy in patients whose visceral encroachment contraindicates the operation. When they are employed as an alternative to adrenalectomy, the patient should be admitted to the hospital and given cortisone therapy initially at high dose, together with intravenous 5-fluorouracil for six days at the rate of 15 mg. per kilogram of body weight. She should then be discharged on low-dose maintenance prednisone (5 mg. twice a day) with 5-fluorouracil (15 mg. per kilogram) given intravenously once a week. This type of joint therapy, although encouraging, is still in an early phase, and it is premature to report statistical response rates.

The possible value of cortisone suppression for five years after prophylactic oophorectomy in the Class B and C cases requires further study.

Chemotherapy*

To many persons unfamiliar with the late course of breast cancer, it does not seem a merciful thing to administer chemotherapy to patients suffering a late exacerbation. No decision in the treatment of this disease requires so much clinical acumen as the choice whether

* We are indebted to Dr. Sidney Farber and his group at the Children's Cancer Research Institute for the entire experience in collaborative chemotherapy.

or not to carry on with additional measures in the late cases. In most of them this decision should be based on the "daily viability" of the patient. If she is up and around, at home, doing her work and still capable of enjoying the world around her, further palliative efforts are justified, not only because of the psychologic support that they give her but more particularly because remarkable results are occasionally obtained.

In the past fifteen years a variety of chemotherapeutic efforts have been made by our group in the treatment of this disease. The most successful by far has been the use of 5-fluorouracil, administered daily for six days at the level of 15 mg. per kilogram of body weight per day in a four-hour intravenous infusion; this is then continued by a weekly syringe injection at about the same dose level with a weekly hemogram. Tables 14 and 15 present data on the chemotherapeutic experience, both with this drug and with thiotepa, its immediate predecessor.

It will be noted that the experience has been extensive, including 124 chemotherapeutic courses, over half of which were major ones (lasting for sixty days) or the sole therapeutic modality. When the drug is used as a terminal measure of desperation, responses are meager, and for this reason there are several entries in Table 14 indicating response rates in "nonterminal courses," which means longer-term therapy in patients with a better outlook.

Table 15 shows the rates and the nature of the complications on chemotherapy. The treatment policy has been to exhibit the drugs at high dosage, the onset of untoward side effects being used as a "cutoff" point. The number of cases in which the drugs were stopped is therefore a measure not so much of the severity of

TABLE 14. *Summary of Chemotherapy for Secondary Disease*

Group	Number of Cases		
Total patients secondary disease			323
Total patients chemotherapy			110/323(34%)
Total episodes chemotherapy			124
Major course (> 60 days or solo)		67	
Minor course (< 60 days or joint)		57	
Total patients positive response			22/110(20%)
Thiotepa, major courses			28
Objective remissions		7/28(25%)	
Objective remissions, nonterminal courses		7/20(35%)	
Remissions > 6 mo., nonterminal courses	2/7		
5-Fluorouracil, major courses			24
Objective remissions		8/24(33%)	
Objective remissions, nonterminal courses		8/20(40%)	
Remissions > 6 mo., nonterminal courses	2/8		
Chemotherapy to manage postoperative exacerbations			30
Objective remissions		8/30(27%)	
With cortisone, to manage exacerbations		50	
Objective remissions	9/50(18%)		

TABLE 15. *Complications of Chemotherapy in Secondary Disease*

Group		Number of Cases	
Total patients receiving			
chemotherapy			110
Complications			46/110(42%)
Leucopenia		24/46(52%)	
Drug stopped		17/24(71%)	
Thiotepa	10		
5-Fluorouracil	4		
Nitrogen mustard	3		
Gastrointestinal		11/46(24%)	
Drug stopped		8/11(78%)	
5-Fluorouracil	5		
Thiotepa	3		
Massive bleeding		4/11	
Total with			
positive response			22/110(20%)
Complications		11/22(50%)	
Drug stopped	4/11(36%)		
Total with			
negative response			88/110(80%)
Complications		35/88(40%)	
Drug stopped	28/35(80%)		
Pancytopenia	19/35(54%)		

complications as of the frequency with which the "cut-off" point was reached. More recent experience has indicated that, in the use of 5-fluorouracil, it is possible to stop the drug for two or three weeks, giving the patient a respite, and then resume the drug at its former dose. This "reinduction" under 5-fluorouracil is a valuable method of managing minor toxic effects.

Our improved experience with chemotherapy has been reflected in the reports of others. Dobson,[121] in 1962, in reviewing the literature on the use of 5-fluorouracil in breast cancer found response rates varying from 21 to 53 per cent. Nevinny,[122] in 1964, reporting for the Eastern Cooperative Group in Solid Tumor Chemotherapy, analyzed the results obtained with 5-

fluorouracil, 5-fluorodeoxyuridine and methotrexate. The onset of response was seen at a median of fifteen days after treatment was initiated, but sometimes as early as seven days, and the greatest number of patients with a response were in the group one to five years after the menopause, with predominantly visceral lesions involving the pleura, lung and liver.

Brennen et al.[123] analyzed the results observed in 124 patients with breast cancer treated with 5-fluorouracil. Regressions and response rates were similar to those reported by the others. Heidelberger and Ansfield[124] reviewed the literature on 5-fluorouracil in cancer chemotherapy up to 1963. In carcinoma of the breast they noted a response rate of 20 to 50 per cent, with an overall average of 32 per cent.

The combined use of 5-fluorouracil with cortisone as an alternative to adrenalectomy and the use of the drug after adrenalectomy have already been mentioned as significant new departures in chemotherapy.

Local Radiotherapy

Of all the measures employed for treatment of the late recurrent disease, local radiotherapy is the most effective and yet the least likely to alter the overall balance between tumor and host, as reflected in duration of life.

Among the 323 patients treated for secondary disease at the Peter Bent Brigham Hospital, 229, or 71 per cent, had one or more episodes of x-ray therapy to local symptomatic areas, usually in bone but sometimes in skin. Thirty-two per cent had treatments three or more times. Of these total treatment episodes, 70 per cent resulted in clear improvement for the patient, of which half the treatments were associated with objective changes and half were symptomatic only. X-ray therapy was given to the fracture area in 8 patients with pathologic fractures. Six were helped by this therapy, and their fractures healed satisfactorily.

8

CONCLUSION

A concerted assault must be made upon the problem of breast cancer because this tumor is a leading cause of death in white women in the United States. It is particularly common in the upper economic classes and in urban populations. In some age and race groups it leads all other causes of death.

Breast cancer seems to arise when genetic and endocrine factors overlap. These genetic and endocrine factors provide important new horizons for the finding and cure of early cases: mothers, sisters, daughters and aunts of patients with this disease are three to ten times as likely as other members of the population to have it.

Normal marriage, pregnancy, childbirth and nursing appear to be associated with a reduced hazard of this disease and to modify its invasive character if it develops.

It appears that a significant decrease in the death rate from this disease would result from improved methods of case finding so as to bring more patients to the surgeon at a time when the high five-year cure rate of 75 to 85 per cent can be realized by operation.

In this favorable setting of localized disease it is extremely unlikely that minor alterations in the surgical protocol will effect any great improvement. Mastectomy combined with dissection of axillary lymph nodes, generally referred to as "standard" or "classic" radical

77

mastectomy, has a record not improved upon by other methods thus far; it possesses, in addition, the unique advantage of providing the pathologist with a large group of axillary lymph nodes for examination. The extent of involvement of these nodes is the single most important factor in prognosis and in the planning of further management. In our opinion the emotional and cosmetic hazards of radical mastectomy have been over-emphasized in the literature.

The likelihood of further axillary or internal-mammary-lymph-node involvement can be gauged from the anatomy of the tumor and its lymph-node metastases; if this involvement shows more than a 30 per cent likelihood, postoperative supervoltage radiotherapy should be given. The position of castration is much less certain, but, like radiotherapy, it is contraindicated in patients with small outer-quadrant lesions in cases in which the axillary lymph nodes are not involved.

For recurrent or metastatic disease, and for patients seen for the first time with advanced local and inoperable tumors, adrenalectomy, in our hands, has won out over other forms of endocrine manipulation as a means of modifying the biologic activity of the tumor. Operative complications are minor, side effects are meager, palliation is significant, duration is impressive, and case selection can produce positive palliative response rates as high as 60 to 70 per cent. Hypophysectomy is as effective as adrenalectomy, but it carries a greater mortality and morbidity.

By contrast, medicinal therapy with sex hormones in the late disease has many unfortunate side effects and gives only transient relief. Minor configurational changes in the sex-hormone structure seem as unlikely to produce any qualitative improvement in results as minor manipulative changes in surgical details of the primary treatment. Corticosteroid therapy, although not entirely free of complications, never produces hypercalcemia — a noteworthy cause of severe complications with both estrogens and androgens. For these reasons, corticosteroid treatment with added 5-fluorouracil has emerged as the most satisfactory alternative to adrenalectomy in patients who are unsuitable for that procedure.

After many years of trial and uncertainty, chemotherapy has emerged with a steady and effective record, 5-fluorouracil being given intravenously. The combination of 5-fluorouracil with adrenalectomy seems to improve the results of both; local radiotherapy to the symptomatic areas is consistently effective for local palliation of disseminated disease.

Until some single solution becomes available to prevent or treat this widespread and devastating disease, a most important step to be taken is that of education. The persons to be educated are the general public, the close female relatives of patients and, finally, the medical profession itself, which, at the time of the first medical contact for the patient, has the best opportunity for cure.

REFERENCES

1. Nathanson, I. T., and Kelley, R. M. Hormonal treatment of cancer. *New Eng. J. Med.* **246**:135-145, 1952.
2. Jessiman, A. G., and Moore, F. D. Carcinoma of breast: study and treatment of patient. *New Eng. J. Med.* **254**:846-853, 900-906, 947-952, 1956.
3. Allen, J. G., and Rigler, S. P. End results from radical mastectomy, with special emphasis on method of follow-up and technique of evaluation. *S. Clin. North America* **42**:1467-1474, 1962.
4. Smithers, D. W. Cancer of breast: study of short survival in early cases and of long survival in advanced cases. *Am. J. Roentgenol.* **80**:740-758, 1958.
5. Devitt, J. E., and Beattie, W. G. Rational treatment of carcinoma of breast. *Ann. Surg.* **160**:71-80, 1964.
6. Bailar, J. C., King, H., and Mason, M. J. *Cancer Rates and Risks.* Washington, D.C.: Government Printing Office, 1964. Publication No. 1148.
7. United States Department of Health, Education and Welfare, Public Health Service. *End Results in Cancer: Report No. 2.* Washington, D.C.: Government Printing Office, 1964. Publication No. 1149.
8. United States Department of Health, Education and Welfare, Public Health Service. *Vital and Health Statistics: Data from the National Health Survey.* Washington, D.C.: Government Printing Office, 1964. Publication No. 1000.
9. Salber, E. J., and Feinleib, M. Breast-feeding in Boston. *Pediatrics* **37**:299-303, 1966.
10. Wainwright, J. M. Comparison of conditions associated with breast cancer in Great Britain and America. *Am. J. Cancer* **15**:2610-2645, 1931.
11. Wood, D. A., and Darling, H. H. Cancer family manifesting multiple occurrences of bilateral carcinoma of breast. *Cancer Research* **3**:509-514, 1943.
12. Penrose, L. S., Mackenzie, H. J., and Karn, M. W. Genetic study of human mammary cancer. *Brit. J. Cancer* **2**:168-176, 1948.
13. Morse, D. P. Hereditary aspect of breast cancer in mother and daughter. *Cancer* **4**:745-748, 1951.
14. Woolf, C. M. *Investigations on Genetic Aspects of Carcinoma of the Stomach and Breast.* Berkeley: Univ. of California Press, 1955.

15. Oliver, C. P. Studies on human cancer families. *Ann. New York Acad. Sc.* **71**:1198-1212, 1957-1958.

16. Anderson, V. E., Goodman, H. O., and Reed, S. C. *Variables Related to Human Breast Cancer: A study from the Dight Institute of Human Genetics.* 172 pp. Minneapolis: Univ. of Minnesota Press, 1958.

17. Macklin, M. T. Comparison of number of breast-cancer deaths observed in relatives of breast-cancer patients and number expected on basis of mortality rates. *J. Nat. Cancer Inst.* **22**:927-951, 1959.

18. Lilienfeld, A. M. Epidemiology of breast cancer. *Cancer Research* **23**:1503-1513, 1963.

19. Gregg, W. I. Galactorrhea after contraceptive hormones. *New Eng. J. Med.* **274**:1432, 1966.

20. Kaufman, R. J., Rothschild, E. O., Escher, G. C., and Myers, W. P. L. Hypercalcemia in mammary carcinoma following administration of progestational agent. *J. Clin. Endocrinol. & Metab.* **24**:1235-1243, 1964.

21. MacMahon, B., and Feinleib, M. Breast cancer in relation to nursing and menopausal history. *J. Nat. Cancer Inst.* **24**:733-753, 1960.

22. Abramson, D. J. 857 Breast biopsies as outpatient procedure: delayed mastectomy in 41 malignant cases. *Ann. Surg.* **163**:478-483, 1966.

23. Haagensen, C. D., et al. Treatment of early mammary carcinoma: cooperative international study. *Ann. Surg.* **157**:157-161, 1963.

24. Haagensen, C. D., and Cooley, E. Radical mastectomy for mammary carcinoma. *Ann. Surg.* **157**:166-169, 1963.

25. Haagensen, C. D. *Diseases of the Breast.* 751 pp. Philadelphia: Saunders, 1956.

26. Byrd, B. F., Jr., Burch, J. C., Stephenson, S. E., Jr., and Nelson, I. A. Effect on survival of certain variables in breast cancer. *Ann. Surg.* **149**:807-814, 1959.

27. Moore, T. C., Judd, D. R., and Moore, W. C. Carcinoma of breast in Middletown, U.S.A. *Surg., Gynec. & Obst.* **107**:433-441, 1958.

28. Breslow, L. Epidemiologic considerations in breast cancer. In *Fifth National Cancer Conference Proceedings.* 764 pp. Philadelphia: Lippincott, 1964. Pp. 125-132.

29. Butcher, H. R. Effectiveness of radical mastectomy for mammary cancer: analysis of mortalities by method of probits. *Ann. Surg.* **154**:383-396, 1961.

30. Guttman, R. J. Radiotherapy in treatment of primary operable carcinoma of breast with proved lymph node metastases: approach and results. *Am. J. Roentgenol.* **89**:58-63, 1963.

31. Miller, E. B. 5 Year review of carcinoma of breast: analysis according to Columbia Classification. *Ann. Surg.* **163**:629-633, 1966.

32. McWhirter, R. Simple mastectomy and radiotherapy in treatment of breast cancer. *Brit. J. Radiol.* **28**:128-139, 1955.

33. Ackerman, L. V. Evaluation of treatment of cancer of breast at University of Edinburgh (Scotland) under direction of Dr. Robert McWhirter. *Cancer* **8**:883-887, 1955.

34. Crile, G., Jr. Results of simplified treatment of breast cancer. *Surg., Gynec. & Obst.* **118**:517-523, 1964.

35. Crile, G., Jr. Metastases from involved lymph nodes after removal of various primary tumors: evaluation of radical and of simple mastectomy for cancers of breast. *Ann. Surg.* **163**:267-271, 1966.

36. Urban, J. S. Personal communication.

37. Urban, J. A., and Farrow, H. Long term results of internal mammary lymph node excision for breast cancer. *Acta, Union internat. Contre Cancer* **19**:1551-1554, 1963.

38. Urban, J. A. Surgical excision of internal mammary nodes for breast cancer. *Brit. J. Surg.* **51**:209-212, 1964.

39. Kaae, S., and Johansen, H. Breast cancer: comparison of results of simple mastectomy with postoperative roentgen irradiation by McWhirter method with those of extended radical mastectomy. *Acta radiol.* Supp. **188**:155-161, 1959.

40. Guttman, R. J. Survival and results after 2 million volt irradiation in treatment of primary operable carcinoma of breast with proved positive internal mammary and/or highest axillary nodes. *Cancer* **15**:383-386, 1962.

41. Hickey, R. C., Kerr, H. D., Tidrick, R. T., Elkins, H. B., and Wieben, E. E. Cancer of breast, 1661 patients: considerations in future therapy. *Arch. Surg.* **73**:654-660, 1956.

42. Smith, G. V., and Smith, O. W. Carcinoma of breast: results, evaluation of x-radiation, and relation of age and surgical castration to length of survival. *Surg., Gynec. & Obst.* **97**:508-516, 1953.

43. Lewison, E. F., and Smith, R. T. Results of breast cancer treatment at Johns Hopkins Hospital, 1946-1950: comparative results and discussion of survival in relation to treatment. *Surgery* **53**:644-656, 1963.

44. Butcher, H. R., Jr., Seaman, W. B., Eckert, C., and Saltzstein, S. Assessment of radical mastectomy and postoperative irradiation therapy in treatment of mammary cancer. *Cancer* **17**:480-485, 1964.

45. Robbins, G. F., Lucas, J. C., Jr., Fracchia, A. A., Farrow, J. H., and Chu, F. C. H. Evaluation of postoperative prophylactic radiation therapy in breast cancer. *Surg., Gynec. & Obst.* **122**:979-982, 1966.

46. Guttman, R. J. Personal communication.

47. Dao, T. L., and Kovaric, J. Incidence of pulmonary and skin metastases in women with breast cancer who received postoperative irradiation. *Surgery* **52**:203-212, 1962.

48. Pearson, O. H., West, C. D., Hollander, V. P., and Escher, G. C. Alterations in calcium metabolism in patients with osteolytic tumors. *J. Clin. Endocrinol. & Metab.* **12**:926, 1952.

49. Jessiman, A. G. Tumour autonomy in carcinoma of breast: problem of recognition of hormone-stimulated tumour. In *Endocrine Aspects of Breast Cancer: Proceedings of a Conference held at the University of Glasgow, 8th to 10th of July, 1957*. Edited by A. P. Currie and C. F. W. Illingworth. Edinburgh: Livingston, 1958. Pp. 77-88.

50. Emerson, K., Jr., and Jessiman, A. G. Hormonal influences on growth and progression of cancer: tests for hormone dependency in mammary and prostatic cancer. *New Eng. J. Med.* **254**:252-258, 1956.

51. Kennedy, B. J., Mielke, P. W., Jr., and Fortuny, I. E. Therapeutic castration versus prophylactic castration in breast cancer. *Surg., Gynec. & Obst.* **118**:524-540, 1964.

52. Kennedy, B. J., and Fortuny, I. E. Therapeutic castration in treatment of advanced breast cancer. *Cancer* **17**:1197-1202, 1964.

53. Nissen-Meyer, R. Prophylactic endocrine treatment in carcinoma of breast. *Clin. Radiol.* **15**:152-160, 1964.

54. Paterson, R., and Russell, M. H. Clinical trials in malignant disease. III. Breast cancer: evaluation of post-operative radiotherapy. *J. Fac. Radiologists* **10**:175-180, 1959.

55. Dealy, J. B. Personal communication.

56. Noer, R. J. Adjuvant chemotherapy: Thio-Tepa with radical mastectomy in treatment of breast cancer. *Am. J. Surg.* **106**:405-412, 1963.

57. Berg, J. W., and Robbins, G. F. Factors influencing short and long term survival of breast cancer patients. *Surg., Gynec. & Obst.* **122**:1311-1316, 1966.

58. Egan, R. L. Mammography: report on 2000 studies. *Surgery* **53**:291-302, 1963.

59. Gershon-Cohen, J., Berger, S. M., and Isard, H. J. Mammography. *Obst. & Gynec.* **27**:102-106, 1966.

60. Witten, D. M., and Thurber, D. L. Mammography as routine screening examination for detecting breast cancer. *Am. J. Roentgenol.* **92**:14-20, 1964.

61. Byrne, R. N., Bringhurst, L. S., and Gershon-Cohen, J. Postoperative detection of cancer by periodic mammography of remaining breast. *Surg., Gynec. & Obst.* **115**:282-286, 1962.

62. Donegan, W. L., Perez-Mesa, C. M., and Watson, F. R. Biostatistical study of locally recurrent breast carcinoma. *Surg., Gynec. & Obst.* **122**:529-540, 1966.

63. Sommers, S. C., and Teloh, H. A. Ovarian stromal hyperplasia in breast cancer. *Arch. Path.* **53**:160-166, 1952.

64. Nissen-Meyer, R., and Sanner, F. Excretion of oestrone, pregnanediol and pregnanetriol in breast cancer patients. I. Excretion after spontaneous menopause. *Acta endocrinol.* **44**:325-333, 1963.

65. Nissen-Meyer, R., and Sanner, F. Excretion of oestrone, pregnanediol and pregnanetriol in breast cancer patients. II. Effect of ovariectomy, ovarian irradiation and corticosteroids. *Acta endocrinol.* **44**:334-345, 1963.

66. Nissen-Meyer, R. Castration as part of primary treatment for operable female breast cancer: statistical evaluation of clinical results. *Acta radiol.* Supp. **249**:1-133, 1965.

67. Castellanos, H., Fairgrieve, J., O'Morchoe, P. J., and Moore, F. D. Corticotropin stimulation of urethral cornification: measure of adrenal estrogen capacity in carcinoma of breast. *J.A.M.A.* **184**: 295-302, 1963.

68. Kleinfeld, G., Haagensen, C. D., and Cooley, E. Age and menstrual status as prognostic factors in carcinoma of breast. *Ann. Surg.* **157**:600-605, 1963.

69. Smithers, D. W., Rigby-Jones, P., Galton, D. A. G., and Payne, P. M. Cancer of breast: review. *Brit. J. Radiol.* Supp. **4**:1-90, 1952.

70. Smith, O. W., and Emerson, K., Jr. Urinary estrogens and related compounds in postmenopausal women with mammary cancer: effect of cortisone treatment. *Proc. Soc. Exper. Biol. & Med.* **85**: 264-267, 1954.

71. Fracchia, A. A., Randall, H. T., and Farrow, J. H. The results of adrenalectomy in advanced breast cancer in 500 consecutive patients. *Surg., Gynec. & Obst.* **125**:747-756, 1967.

72. Bulbrook, R. D., Greenwood, F. C., and Hayward, J. L. Selection of breast-cancer patients for adrenalectomy or hypophysectomy by determination of urinary 17-hydroxycorticosteroids and aetiocholanolone. *Lancet* **1**:1154-1157, 1960.

73. Atkins, H., et al. Urinary steroid estimations in prediction of response to adrenalectomy or hypophysectomy. *Lancet* **2**:1133-1136, 1964.

74. Hayward, J. L., and Bulbrook, R. D. Value of urinary steroid estimations in prediction of response to adrenalectomy or hypophysectomy. *Cancer Research* **25**:1129-1134, 1965.

75. Bulbrook, R. D., and Hayward, J. L. Possibility of predicting response of patients with early breast cancer to subsequent endocrine ablation. *Cancer Research* **25**:1135-1139, 1965.

76. Jantet, G., Crocker, D. W., Shiraki, M., and Moore, F. D. Adrenal suppression in disseminated carcinoma of breast. I. Effect on adrenal morphology of hypophysectomy and corticosteroid treatment. *New Eng. J. Med.* **269**:1-7, 1963.

77. Wilson, R. E., et al. Adrenal structure and function in advanced carcinoma of breast. II. Relation of steroid excretion to adrenal morphology and outcome of adrenalectomy, with description of new discriminant function. *J.A.M.A.* **199**:474-482, 1967.

78. Wilson, R. E., Jessiman, A. G., and Moore, F. D. Severe exacerbation of cancer of breast, after oöphorectomy and adrenalectomy: report of four cases. *New Eng. J. Med.* **258**:312-317, 1958.

79. Ray, B. Hypophysectomy as palliative treatment for disseminated carcinoma. *J.A.M.A.* (in press).

80. Jessiman, A. G., Matson, D. D., and Moore, F. D. Hypophysectomy in treatment of breast cancer. *New Eng. J. Med.* **261**:1199-1207, 1959.

81. MacDonald, I. Endocrine ablation in disseminated mammary carcinoma. *Surg., Gynec. & Obst.* **115**:215-222, 1962.

82. Dingman, J. F., et al. Residual neurohypophyseal function in hypophysectomized man. *New Eng. J. Med.* **260**:997-1001, 1959.

83. Little, B., et al. Hypophysectomy during pregnancy in patient with cancer of breast: case report with hormone studies. *J. Clin. Endocrinol. & Metab.* **18**:425-443, 1958.

84. Volkman, A., Crocker, D. W., Jessiman, A. G., and Emerson, E., Jr. Clinicopathologic correlation of effect of hypophysectomy in seven female patients with advanced carcinoma of breast. *Am. J. Surg.* **103**:415-423, 1962.

85. Edelstyn, G. A., Gleadhill, C. A., and Lyons, A. R. Hypophysectomy and breast cancer. *Lancet* **1**:1211, 1966.

86. Forrest, A. P. M., et al. Radio-active implantation of pituitary. *Brit. J. Surg.* **47**:61-70, 1959.

87. Forrest, A. P. M., and Stewart, H. J. Unpublished data.

88. Forrest, A. P. M. Personal communication.

89. Delarue, N. C. Adrenalectomy in management of metastatic mammary carcinoma: final evaluation of 80 cases. *Canad. J. Surg.* **4**:22-34, 1960.

90. Kambouris, A. A., Saltzstein, H. C., and Scheinberg, S. Bilateral adrenalectomy for advanced breast cancer: review of literature and analysis of twenty-five cases. *Am. J. Surg.* **102**:651-656, 1961.

91. Mye, G. L., Jr., and Neal, W., Jr. Bilateral adrenalectomy for advanced mammary cancer: 9-year review of 84 cases. *Am. Surgeon* **31**:621-624, 1965.

92. Daicoff, G. R., Harmon, R., and Van Prohaska, J. Effect of adrenalectomy on mammary carcinoma. *Arch. Surg.* **85**:800-807, 1962.

93. Falconer, M. A. Relative values of surgical hypophysectomy and of bilateral adrenalectomy with oophorectomy in treatment of metastatic breast cancer. *Proc. Roy. Soc. Med.* **53**:637, 1960.

94. Nelsen, T. S., and Dragstedt, L. R. Adrenalectomy and oophorectomy for breast cancer. *J.A.M.A.* **175**:379-383, 1961.

95. Alrich, E. M., and Brown, L. B. Adrenalectomy for far-advanced breast carcinoma: report of sixteen cases. *Virginia M. Monthly* **86**:524-527, 1959.

96. Krieger, H., Abbott, W. E., Storaasli, J. P., and Friedell, L. Combined therapy for palliation of metastatic carcinoma of breast. *Bull. Soc. Internat. Chir.* **19**:515-525, 1960.

97. Dao, T. L., and Tan, E. Comparative evaluation of adrenalectomy and androgen in advanced mammary carcinoma. *Cancer Chemotherapy Rep.* **16**:309-315, 1962.

98. Biswanger, L. T., Averbook, B. D., Weber, R. A., and Barker, W. F. Adrenalectomy for metastatic carcinoma of breast. *West. J. Surg.* **68**:128-134, 1960.

99. Atkins, H. J. B., et al. Adrenalectomy and hypophysectomy for advanced cancer of breast. *Lancet* **1**:1148-1153, 1960.

100. Parsons, W. H., Blackshear, S. G., and Lee, S. S. Total adrenalectomy for advanced carcinoma of breast: with report of twenty-five additional cases. *South. M. J.* **53**:941-944, 1960.

101. Dao, T. L., Tan, E., and Brooks, V. Comparative evaluation of adrenalectomy and cortisone in treatment of advanced mammary carcinoma. *Cancer* **14**:1259-1265, 1961.

102. Byron, R. L., Jr., et al. Bilateral adrenalectomy in advanced breast cancer. *Surgery* **52**:725-732, 1962.

103. McLaughlin, J. S., Hull, H. C., Oda, F., and Buxton, R. W. Metastatic carcinoma of male breast: remission by adrenalectomy. *Ann. Surg.* **162**:9-14, 1965.

104. Crocker, D. W., Fairgrieve, J., O'Morchoe, P. J. O., and Moore, F. D. Adrenal cortical suppression in rat: effects of hydrocortisone with and without desoxycorticosterone acetate. *J. S. Research* **4**:562-566, 1964.

105. Hall, T. C., and Wilson, R. E. Safe and effective method of administering 5-fluorouracil to adrenalectomized patients. *Surg., Gynec. & Obst.* **123**:978-982, 1966.

106. Jessiman, A. G., Emerson, K., Jr., Shah, R. C., and Moore, F. D. Hypercalcemia in carcinoma of breast. *Ann. Surg.* **157**:377-393, 1963.

107. Kleinfeld, G. Acute fatal hypercalcemia: complication in estrogen therapy of metastatic breast cancer. *J.A.M.A.* **181**:1137, 1962.

108. Sackner, M. A., Spivack, A. P., and Balian, L. J. Hypocalcemia in presence of osteoblastic metastases. *New Eng. J. Med.* **262**:173-176, 1960.

109. Ehrlich, M., Goldstein, M., and Heinemann, H. O. Hypocalcemia, hypoparathyroidism, and osteoblastic metastases. *Metabolism* **12**:516-526, 1963.

110. Hall, T. C., Griffiths, C. T., and Petranek, J. R. Hypocalcemia — unusual metabolic complication of breast cancer. *New Eng. J. Med.* **275**:1474-1477, 1966.

111. Emerson, K., Jr., Muller, J., de Souza, A., and Loutfi, G. Paradoxical response of metastatic breast cancer to 17-ethyl-19-nortestosterone. *Ann. Int. Med.* **55**:742-748, 1961.

112. Myers, W. P. L., West, C. D., Pearson, O. H., and Karnofsky, D. A. Androgen-induced exacerbation of breast cancer measured by calcium excretion: conversion of androgen to estrogen as possible underlying mechanism. *J.A.M.A.* **161**:127-131, 1956.

113. Steinach, E., and Kun, H. Transformation of male sex hormones into substance with action of female hormone. *Lancet* **2**:845, 1937.

114. Hoskins, W. H., Coffman, J. R., Koch, F. C., and Kenyon, A. T. Effect of testosterone proprionate on urinary excretion of androgens and estrogens in eunuchoidism. *Endocrinology* **24**:702-710, 1939.

115. Dorfman, R. I., and Hamilton, J. B. Urinary excretion of estrogenic substances after administration of testosterone proprionate to humans. *Endocrinology* **25**:33-38, 1939.

116. Dao, T. L., and Nemoto, T. Evaluation of adrenalectomy and androgen in disseminated mammary carcinoma. *Surg., Gynec. & Obst.* **121**:1257-1262, 1965.
117. Rosoff, C. B. Hormonal therapy of breast cancer: summary of experience with newer steroids. In Conference on the Biological Activities of Steroids in Relation to Cancer, Vergennes, Vermont, 1959. *Biological Activities of Steroids in Relation to Cancer: Proceedings of a Conference Sponsored by the Cancer Chemotherapy National Service Center, National Cancer Institute, National Institutes of Health, United States Department of Health, Education, and Welfare.* Edited by G. Pincus and E. P. Vollmer. 530 pp. New York: Academic Press, 1960. Pp. 363-383.
118. Smith, O. W., and Emerson, K., Jr. Urinary estrogens and related compounds in postmenopausal women with mammary cancer: effect of cortisone treatment. *Proc. Soc. Exper. Biol. & Med.* **85**: 264-267, 1954.
119. Jessiman, A. G., and Moore, F. D. *Carcinoma of the Breast: The study and treatment of the patient.* 135 pp. Boston: Little, Brown, 1956.
120. Sherlock, P., and Hartmann, W. H. Adrenal steroids and pattern of metastases of breast cancer. *J.A.M.A.* **181**:313-317, 1962.
121. Dobson, L. Treatment of recurrent or metastatic breast cancer with emphasis on use of 5-fluorouracil. *Am. J. Surg.* **104**:143-154, 1962.
122. Nevinny, H. B. Comparative study of 5-fluorouracil (FU), 5-fluorodeoxyuridine (FUDR) and methotrexate (MTX) in patients with advanced cancer. *Proc. Am. A. Cancer Research* **5**:47, 1964.
123. Brennan, M. J., et al. Critical analysis of 594 cancer patients treated with 5-fluorouracil. In International Symposium on Chemotherapy of Cancer. *Proceedings of the Symposium, Lugano, 28th April to 1st May, 1964: Organized by the Swiss Academy of Medical Sciences and sponsored by F. Hoffmann-LaRoche & Co. Ltd.* Edited by P. A. Plattner. 324 pp. Amsterdam: C. Elsevier Pub. Co., 1964. Pp. 118-149.
124. Heidelberger, C., and Ansfield, F. J. Experimental and clinical use of fluorinated pyrimidines in cancer chemotherapy. *Cancer Research* **23**:1226-1243, 1963.